You Can
Get Well

You Can Get Well

by
Adelle Davis, A.B., M.S.
Nutritionist

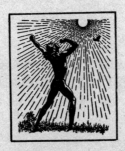

Published and Distributed by
BENEDICT LUST PUBLICATIONS
Box 404 • **New York 10156**

Dedicated to a person whose name I do not know, who lived I know not when, but who first said, "An ounce of prevention is worth a pound of cure."

FOREWORD

Adelle Davis reminds me of an interesting aunt who comes to visit. Her visits are always anticipated pleasurably in the expectation that we'll learn something new about ourselves and how we function.

She knows her subject. And, unlike so many in her field, she is able to EXPLAIN IT TO OTHERS. Her style is clear, readable, casual, conversational, yet meaty with scientific facts, simply told.

Raised on an Indiana farm, she took her professional training at Purdue University and the University of California. Later she did post graduate work at Columbia University and UCLA. She earned her degree of Master of Science at the University of Southern California Medical School. After she completed training as a dietitian at Bellevue Hospital, she became Nutritional Consultant and Supervisor of Health Education in the Public Schools in New York City.

Millions of her books have been sold. She helped hundreds of thousands of people on the road to better health. Her daily contact with people and their health problems makes her book meet **your** problem, discussed in your **language**.

Not very long ago, it was widely accepted that your diet had little or nothing to do with your health. Thanks are due to Adelle Davis for playing a key role in correcting this fallacy.

New York, N.Y.   John Lust
September, 1975

Marie and I had talked diet all afternoon.

"I wanted to ask you," she said, "which food is . . ."

"Please, Marie," I interrupted, "I'm sick of talking diet."

She turned quickly, looking at me in astonishment.

"I've a friend who's a radio engineer," I explained. "He's an expert, and I remember hearing him say that no matter where he went, people always made him talk radios. Said he never goes to visit anyone that a radio isn't on the blink and he is asked to fix it." I smiled drily. "I'm in the same boat. I talk diet to patients, doctors, radio listeners, women's clubs, and men's luncheons. You heard the conversation at May's house. At Miller's supper party the other night, we talked about diet to improve eyesight. Yesterday Cynthia, Walter, and I were having a bit to eat, and believe it or not, we talked about diet to grow hair."

"It's because you're so enthusiastic and interested in the subject," Marie said comfortingly. "I've an idea. Write a book about these talks and conversations. People would learn more that way than by wading through hundreds of pages of dry texts."

The longer I thought about her suggestion, the better I liked it. Others seemed to like it too.

This book is the result, written because people are interested in the preservation of their health and because progress along the road between research findings and common knowledge, applied to ones' daily life, is slow. The conversations actually took place, essentially as they have been given. Many of the characters have requested that I use their own names; other names are changed, the substitutes largely chosen by the people themselves. In every case history, the names used are fictitious. I was surprised to find that people are usually flattered to be put into a book. In fact, my neighbor's young daughter said, after she had read part of the manuscript, "If I ask you enough questions, will you make me a character in your book?"

Adelle Davis

CONTENTS

ARE YOU UP TO DATE?

Fred lay in a high hospital bed and was almost as white as the sheets. He had lost weight, and his forehead looked narrower and longer. I was sitting in an easy chair near his bed, talking to him.

"I've always taken my health for granted," he said. "I've never been sick before. So I somehow thought I never would be. Now I'd give everything I possess for my health. It's the only thing that really matters. Other people must feel the same way I always have. They should be made to understand how important health is, before it's too late. That's your business. Bring their ideas up to date."

I smiled, remembering Fred's attitude only a few weeks before. "And what if they don't want to be brought up to date?"

"But they do!" His tone reminded me of the old Fred. "This is a progressive age. Why, people are so proud of being progressive that they dislike being out of date in the slightest thing."

"Yes, I know." There was sarcasm in my voice. "But these same people are *eating out of date*."

Fred looked surprised.

"In hundreds of laboratories all over the world, scientists are experimenting to find the cause of ill health, the first beginnings of disease. They've already proved that many diseases can be prevented, and sometimes it seems that almost every illness is unnecessary if prevention could be started early enough."

"Why isn't the public told about it?" Fred demanded intolerantly.

"It's true that people sometimes don't learn how a disease can be prevented until years after research has been done. Even when information does become generally known, it's less often accepted and applied than other things which may have no direct influence on one's happiness. Too often people's minds are closed."

He gave a wry smile. "I'm afraid I've been guilty of that."

"Fred, as simple as good nutrition is, its daily application as a means of building radiant health and preventing disease is still rare. Nutrition is nothing more than intelligently planned

11

health, but people don't understand that. It seems to be human nature to think, just as you did, that the other person will always be the one to become ill. The barest suggestion of heart disease makes them say, 'My heart's strong. I'll never have heart trouble.' Their reactions to other abnormalities are much the same.''

He seemed thoughtful. "You see, that's called wishful thinking. People want to have good health. They convince themselves they always will have, even though they do nothing to promote it." After a moment's hesitation he added, "Knowing you can't live makes many things seem of little consequence. The things I thought were important weren't important, even then. The really important things, I overlooked. Tell everyone that health is extremely important."

We sat in silence. I kept thinking how important health really is, not for itself, but in order that we can give our full energies to work and to play and to the many rich values life has to offer us.

EAT FIVE OR SIX TIMES DAILY

Gail and I were tired from shopping; our husbands were weary after their day's work.

"I'm hungry enough to eat a horse," Gail exclaimed abruptly. "I'm going to have something to eat even if it isn't mealtime."

"People should eat something between meals," I answered.

Ed nodded. "I read in an article that people had more pep and did better work if they ate five or six times a day. Persons who ate five times a day turned out twice as much work as those who ate only two meals. They felt more rested and made fewer mistakes. No one asked them to work harder, either. Persons who didn't eat between meals became tired and irritable and weren't efficient."

When breakfast has been early, have fruit, fruit juice, raw carrots, or milk in the middle of the morning.

Eat a small meal in the afternoon: cheese and crackers; fruit; banana and milk; fruit or vegetable juices.

If you are doing hard physcial work or taking vigorous exercise, eat somewhat heavier midmeals: a peanut-butter or cheese sandwich; yogurt with cinnamon and blackstrap molasses; dried fruit; or a milk drink.

Give children small midmeals at definite times not later than 3 hours before the next meal: sandwiches of whole-wheat bread; fresh or dried fruit; milk or yogurt.

When dinner is served early, have a light meal rich in calcium before retiring: milk, buttermilk, a milk drink, yogurt, or cheese and crackers.

Avoid eating candy, cookies, cake, soft drinks, or other concentrated sweets between meals; eating concentrated sugar overstimulates insulin flow which causes the blood sugar to drop below normal and fatigue to increase.

Do not increase total food intake unless weight is below normal; subtract food for midmeals from regular meals.

One of the chief reasons for overweight is failure to eat between meals. If you are reducing, take the edge off your appetite by eating midmeals 1 to 1½ hours before the next meal; have a midmeal of raw vegetables, tomato juice, skim milk, or a heaping tablespoon of brewers' yeast stirred into a glass of water.

YOU CAN HAVE AN ADEQUATE DIET AT LOW COST

"So you know the Taylors!" we both exclaimed at once.

Betty recovered her surprise first. "I've never seen any family change like that before. When I first knew them, invariably someone was sick. Then they seemed to be getting along all right, and the first thing I knew, each was looking the picture of health."

"Those children's health means more to Mr. Taylor than anything else in the world," I answered. "All I had to do was to say the children should have certain vitamins and minerals, and tell Mr. Taylor what foods furnished them. As I see it, Betty, anyone's health isn't a matter of dollars and cents, but of intelligence and planning, often of pluck and hard work, prompted by the conviction of the value of health. And the reward certainly justifies the effort."

When the buget is limited, use powered skim milk which can be purchased from dairies. Prepare reconstructed milk by combining ½ cup of the powder with 1 quart of water; use in baking and in making soups, custards, puddings, milk drinks.

Purchase blackstrap molasses, extremely rich in calcium, iron, and many B vitamins, directly from molasses companies or from any bakery supply house. Stir into milk or yogurt, use for sweetening "caramel" puddings, ice creams, or custards; make into gingerbread and molasses cookies.

Obtain 100 per cent whole-wheat flour, wheat germ, unground wheat, soybeans, and similar products in bulk directly from the flour mill. Serve cooked unground wheat and whole buckwheat as a cereal or a meat substitute, preparing them with meat as you would rice, macaroni, or noodles. Grind cooked soybeans, season well, and make into meatloaf and patties. Get acquainted with soy grits; add to cereals, custards, puddings, cookies.

Margarin is nutritionally equivalent to summer butter; use it instead of butter; use evaporated milk instead of cream.

Purchase inexpensive cuts of meat free from fat and bone: liver, heart, brain, kidneys, tongue; respect the lowly hot dog. Prepare your own liverwurst. Use the cheaper varieties of fish and sea food: mussels, canned mackerel, inexpensive fresh fish.

Plan your garden and plant fruit trees to produce vitamins and minerals; get acquainted with all varieties of vegetables.

Can foods in season.

If purchasing fish-liver oil or vitamin concentrates, select potency and price rather than brand names.

KEEP YOUR EYES SPARKLING

Glen glanced around to see if anyone else was going to speak. "Weren't you saying that 50 per cent of the people in the country were partially night blind, and that some tests showed that those on relief were sometimes as high as 75 per cent?"

"Several studies have shown that," I answered, "especially the work of Dr. Jeans and Dr. Zentmire in Iowa. They also found

14

that city children had much poorer vision than country children. Jeghers points out that people quite low in vitamin A considered themselves perfectly healthy. When questioned, however, many complained of difficulty in sewing or reading at night unless the light was brilliant, of dancing figures and specks on the page, of glittering images, of nervousness and fatigue resulting from even slight use of their eyes, and even of muscular twitching of the eyelids. The hopeful part is, though, that it can be cleared up in a few days if large amounts of vitamin A are eaten. It need never return if adequate amounts are always supplied in the diet."

"Mother sews and darns a good deal at night," Cynthia said. "She's always complaining of her eyes, but the oculist says there's nothing wrong with them."

"That's true of hundreds of older people," I replied. "When their eyes bother them, they say it's their age and let it go at that. The customary eye examination, unfortunately, does not test for vitamin deficiencies. In almost any trouble with the eyes, it's a good idea to go to a physician who will test the eyes for vitamin A before considering glasses. If that were done, there would be far fewer glasses worn in this country." I thought a moment. "Diet has more to do with the eyes than most people ever dream of. It's one of the places where nutrition really gets its feet on the ground and affects everyone's life personally."

If vitamin A is undersupplied, the eyes become sensitive to light; night vision may be impaired; the eyes become strained easily, and physical fatigue results. If a severe deficiency occurs, the eyelids burn, the eyeballs ache and become sore, the eyes become susceptible to infection.

When vitamin B_2, or riboflavin, is deficient, the eyes become sensitive to light, water easily, and feel as if grains of sand were under the lids; they sometimes become bloodshot; on occasions the lids may burn and become red and swollen; symptoms are exaggerated after the eyes are used. Night vision remains normal, but vision is difficult in dim light.

If you feel more comfortable wearing dark glasses, your intake of vitamins A and/or B_2 is probably low.

To maintain normal vision, be sure that your daily diet supplies at least 10,000 units of vitamin A and 3 milligrams of riboflavin. Vitamin A is absorbed best when taken directly afrer meals. To prevent urinary loss, no more than 3 milligrams of riboflavin should be taken at one time. Increase the amount of each vitamin whenever you expect to use your eyes for long hours or in bright or dim lights.

When definite deficiencies exist, physicians often recommend as much as 150,000 units of vitamin A and 20 milligrams of riboflavin be taken daily for 3 or 4 weeks. Vitamin E must be adequate before vitamin A can be utilized.

The B vitamin, biotin, helps to protect your eyes against infections; see that your biotin intake is adequate by generous use of wheat germ, brewers' yeast, liver, blackstrap molasses, and other foods rich in the B vitamins.

Nearsightedness can be produced in animals by a diet deficient in calcium and vitamin D; farsightedness results from poor muscle tone, caused largely by protein deficiency.

Cataracts can be produced in animals by lack of any of the three nutrients: riboflavin, or vitamin B_2; ascorbic acid, or vitamin C; and the amino acid, tryptophane, supplied by proteins such as milk, eggs, cheese, and meat. Cataracts in humans have often disappeared following a diet rich in these nutrients.

MODERN COOKING
BUILDS HEALTH AND IMPROVES FLAVOR

Cynthia stood dusting the mantel, carefully going over each photograph and knick-knack.

I dropped into the worn leather chair.

"Most foods are about 70 to 90 per cent water, and that's plenty to cook them in if one has equipment which will prevent steam—and incidentally flavors—from escaping. A heavy metal is a much better conductor of heat than water is. The cooking is done from the sides and top of scientific utensils, and therefore less fuel is needed; cooking time is shorter, and thus fewer vitamins are destroyed. Close-fitting lids prevent air from coming in to harm the vitamins too; there's no water to dissolve out either minerals or vitamins, and none to be thrown away later. Scientific utensils are really bake ovens which can be used on top of the stove. The method is very similar to that of the old fireless cooker; after the utensil is hot, very little heat is needed to finish the cooking. Foods can cook at much lower temperatures than most people seem to think.''

Cynthia sat down in the walnut rocker. ''Isn't aluminum supposed to be harmful?''

''There's aluminum in the body. Also in bodies of animals which have never eaten from aluminum utensils. Instead of being dangerous, it may be essential to health, as some scientists think. Quite large amounts have been fed or injected into people and have caused no harmful results.''

''I'll admit foods cooked without water taste better.''

''Dr. Okey of the University of California made a study of cooking methods at a school for blind children. The youngsters didn't like vegetables, but when the foods were prepared properly —not soaked before cooking, not overcooked, not reheated, or prepared hours before serving time—they ate large amounts and asked for more. Even during a short period, the children showed greater gains in weight, and their general health improved, although the same amount of money was spent on food and the selection was the same. Any mother whose family won't eat vegetables should see if there isn't something wrong with her cooking methods.''

Cynthia slowly shook her head. ''It's hard to realize that enough food value is lost to make such a difference in health.''

''Correct cooking methods can cause a tremendous improvement in your health. A tiny loss, day after day, can add up to a significant loss in the course of a few months, and mean the difference between poor health and excellent health in a few years.''

Wash all firm vegetables and fruits as soon as they are brought into the house; dry root vegetables with an old Turkish towel; shake water from leafy vegetables by whirling in a cheesecloth bag; put into a covered refrigerator pan, or hydrater; chill as quickly as possible.

Avoid soaking in all forms; wash foods as quickly as possible, and put them on a tray in a covered refrigerator pan; instead

17

of soaking vegetables to freshen them, keep water under the tray; above all, avoid boiling vegetables, which is soaking at its worst.

Cook vegetables by the "waterless" method or by steaming, sautéing, broiling, or low-temperature frying; do not boil.

Use cooking utensils with tight-fitting lids. Avoid cooking in glass; light brings about rapid destruction of riboflavin, or vitamin B_2. Since copper causes instantaneous destruction of ascorbic acid, or vitamin C, discard all cooking utensils which contain copper; discard knives which are not chrome plated, stainless steel, or plastic; iron frying pans and Dutch ovens; rusty strainers, colanders, graters, stirring spoons.

Except for searing, cook all meats at low temperatures. Add 1 or 2 tablespoons of vinegar to stews and braised meats containing bone in order to dissolve calcium into the gravy.

Avoid peeling vegetables whenever possible. Chop vegetables as little as possible unless thoroughly chilled. Start cooking vegetables in preheated utensils or preheated oven; heat through as quickly as possible; serve as soon as tender. Use leftover vegetables in salads to avoid reheating. Heat canned foods in their own liquid.

Save all edible vegetable parings, leftover salads, table scraps, and any water left from steaming for making soup stock; add vinegar, tomatoes, or other acid to all soups in order to dissolve calcium from the bones into the stock.

If citrus juice is to be squeezed before being served, keep air tight in a closed container in the refrigerator; transfer to smaller container when some is used, keeping container so full that no air space is left above juice.

Modernize all recipes before using them; use whole-wheat flour instead of white; substitute wheat germ, rice polish, or soy, peanut, or cottonseed flour for a third or more of the flour called for; add powdered milk, sifting it with the flour; decrease temperature and cooking time when possible.

When preparing dry beans, peas, or similar foods, cook them in the water used for soaking; do not parboil and discard water. Avoid adding soda.

In baking, use baking powder in preference to soda, yeast in preference to baking powder.

HEALTHY HAIR IS BEAUTIFUL HAIR

Some people say that experimental animals should not be given inadequate diets; yet those very people often unknowingly feed their own pets inadequate diets. In fact, they frequently eat even poorer diets themselves and sometimes produce serious diseases in their own bodies. Rarely are their diets lacking in only one nutrient. If people could develop sufficient humility, they could learn from animals so many things which, if applied to themselves, could greatly decrease suffering and increase happiness. Of course there is a difference in species, but the nourishment needed to keep each tissue healthy—heart, lungs, glands, teeth, digestive tract, nerves, hair, all of which are common to both humans and animals—is essentially the same.

By various diets lacking only one nutrient, all types of abnormal hair can be produced in animals; rough hair; coarse hair; oily hair; hair which lacks luster; gray hair, falling hair, or a total absence of hair. The same conditions may be produced in humans.

Probably every nutrient influences the health of the hair.

Hair is made of protein; it is largely made of the sulfur-containing amino acids obtained from eating fish, milk, cheese, meat, and particularly eggs. A protein deficiency reflects itself in slow-growing and thin hair.

Adequate amounts of iron, copper, iodine, and the following B vitamins are essential in maintaining the natural color of hair: pantothenic acid, or calcium pantothenate; para aminobenzoic acid, or paba; and folic acid. Another B vitamin, inositol, may help to maintain hair color. Gray hair at any age, particularly premature gray hair, probably indicates a deficiency of one or more of these nutrients.

The natural color of gray hair has sometimes been restored by an adequate intake of all the anti-gray-hair vitamins. In experimental studies, color restoration has been noted in about 30 per cent of the persons taking pantothenic acid; in 70 per cent of those taking para aminobenzoic acid; no clinical studies have been made of color restoration following the use of folic acid or inositol.

Most marked results in restoration of color to gray hair have come from the liberal use of natural foods supplying B vitamins: brewers' yeast; blackstrap molasses; wheat germ; rice polish; liver; yogurt.

When liberal amounts of yogurt are drunk daily, the yogurt bacteria growing in the intestinal tract apparently synthesize, or produce, inositol and the anti-gray-hair vitamins.

A lack of vitamin A causes the hair to be coarse and lacking in luster; this deficiency may be a causative factor in dandruff formation.

Excessive dandruff and falling hair often indicate poor circulation to the scalp. Make sure that your diet supplies sufficient iodine and B vitamins to maintain normal circulation.

The B vitamin, inositol, appears to prevent baldness; male animals require twice as much of this vitamin as do female animals. Every man who wishes to keep his hair should see that his daily diet contains adequate inositol. The richest sources of this vitamin are whole-wheat breads, brewers' yeast, blackstrap molasses, and wheat germ.

KEEP YOUR RESISTANCE TO INFECTIONS HIGH

Marie backed away from the sink, bent forward, and sneezed several times. "My immunity's low. Guess my antibodies are getting feeble."

"Better go heavy on protein for a while," I said. "Saw the report of a study the other day. People were fed a diet low in protein for only a week. The number of antibodies fell to a tenth that of normal. Can't expect criminals to be captured when you don't feed the police force."

"But I thought vitamin C was the important thing in antibody production."

"The number of antibodies does decrease when you don't get enough C. The vitamin C appears to work almost as antibodies do. When bacteria or any other foreign substances get into the blood, vitamin C seems to combine with them and render them harmless; then the two are excreted in the urine. That's why vitamin C is given as a treatment for so many different things — lead poisoning, all types of allergies, various drug poisonings, and almost any type of infection.''

Adequate rest, sleep, absorption of foods, and good elimination all play a role in helping to prevent infections.

A lack of almost any nutrient may lead to low resistance. Deficiencies of vitamins A, C, biotin, and protein appear to result most quickly in susceptibility to infections.

Studies have shown that few antibodies are produced when protein is undersupplied. To maintain high resistance, estimate the grams of protein you eat daily and make sure that the amount is adequate.

The greatest single cause of colds appears to be contagion; the second, lack of sleep; the third, inadequate diet. Even the most perfect diet will probably not prevent colds entirely.

Frequent colds and colds which hang on invariably indicate that the nutrition is poor. See that your daily diet supplies adequate protein, 100 to 300 milligrams of ascorbic acid, or vitamin C, and 50,000 units or more of vitamin A daily until your resistance is built up.

If you are taking a cold or have a cold, stay in bed. Do not expose others to your infection.

During a cold or any other acute infection, increase protein intake to 80 or more grams daily; drink a quart of milk, have 1 or more eggs, a serving of cottage cheese, and any other proteins desired. Take 100 milligrams of ascorbic acid, preferably in tablet form, every 2 or 3 hours while the infection is severe. Continue adequate protein and 200 or 300 milligrams of ascorbic acid until resistance is high. Avoid drinking large amounts of citrus juices, which may make body fluids so alkaline as to promote the growth of bacteria.

During infections of the mucous membranes, such as colitis and infections of the throat, sinus, mastoid, kidney, bladder, and lungs, 100,000 units or more of vitamin A should be taken daily until resistance is high; 10 to 25 milligrams of vitamin E, or alpha tocopherol, should be obtained to insure efficient utilization of the vitamin A.

Sulfa drugs are effective because they destroy B vitamins required by bacteria; therefore foods rich in the B vitamins should be avoided when sulfa is taken. After the infection has cleared, large amounts of brewers' yeast, wheat germ, liver, and blackstrap molasses should be used to overcome the induced deficiency.

SALT IS REQUIRED FOR HEALTH

I happened to admire a beautiful, hand-wrought tablespoon which lay on the cloth before me.

Elena noticed my interest. "I still have three of them. The only possessions I managed to take when we left Odessa." A far-away look came into her dark eyes. "I had ten then, but I traded the others for salt."

"For salt!" I exclaimed.

"Some evidence indicates your cravings are for foods your body needs most," Glen remarked.

Boris frowned over his tea cup. "I thought salt was bad."

"Did you read about the prospector who died recently on the desert?" Glen asked. "Man at the office knew him. He was a food faddist who wouldn't eat any salt. Look what happened to him."

"Faddists had better keep out of the heat if they want to stay faddists," I remarked.

"That's what caused the deaths the first few years at Boulder Dam," Glen explained to Boris, who looked puzzled.

"So much salt's lost in perspiration that the men died from lack of it," I said. "The problem was first studied in a mine in England where it was extremely hot. The miners complained of continuous exhaustion, of cramps in their legs, back and abdomen. Several died of heat prostration. In spite of the heat, the body temperature of the stricken men was about normal. The more water they drank, the worse the cramps became. Finally the perspiration lost during a shift was collected in big rubber boots, and analysis showed that it sometimes contained as much as four tablespoonfuls—two ounces—of salt. As soon as the men were given salt water to drink, the exhaustion and cramps disappeared, and there were no more deaths."

Do not avoid salt unless advised to do so by your physician.

Unless the weather is unusually warm, let your taste for salt be your guide; salt generously rather than sparingly.

During hot weather, keep salty foods near the drinking water: salty crackers, popcorn, peanuts, potato chips, salty cheeses, pretzels, salted soybeans.

Serve one salty food at each meal during hot weather: salt-cured fish or pork; salty cheeses, sauerkraut, corned beef, or any vegetable or meat to which generous amounts of salt have been added.

If working in extremely high temperatures, take 1 or 2 salt tablets with each glass of liquid.

YOUR THYROID GLAND IS YOUR ACCELERATOR

Cynthia sat down in the big green chair opposite my desk. "Went in for my yearly checkup. Been gaining too easily, haven't any pep, and the worst of it is, can't remember anything. I'll get as far as a door and can't remember what I've started to do."

"Did Dr. Collins tell you to take iodine?"

"Yes. A drop in a glass of water every day for two weeks, then two drops a week to be continued indefinitely."

"Too little iodine prevents the thyroid gland from functioning normally. That's the tiny gland on either side of the windpipe." I placed my fingers on my neck. "The thyroid's like an accelerator in a car; it controls the speed of the engine. A metabolism of minus seventeen shows your engine's pretty sluggish. Zero is normal, and a plus something or other would show the motor is running faster than average."

Cynthia sat relaxed, listening intently.

"A sluggish thyroid allows the heart to beat more slowly than it should. Slow heartbeat causes poor circulation—cold hands and feet, unhealthy hair, skin, and nails. That's probably the reason you're having trouble remembering—poor circulation in the brain. When it's extremely hot, the sluggish blood stream fails to cool the body properly, and you suffer from heat. In mildly hot weather, you probably feel fine."

"That's the kind of weather I like."

"Your iodine-deficient thyroid also causes too little food to be burned in your body—another reason you suffer from cold, lack pep, and gain easily. The same lack of vitality is shown by your low blood pressure and your tendency toward constipation. A small amount of iodine may seem unimportant, but it can make the difference between feeling rotten or being on top of the world."

A slight thyroid deficiency, caused by lack of iodine, can result in overweight, lack of drive and energy, sluggish thinking, low blood pressure, anemia, sensitiveness to cold and heat, and slowed circulation causing cold hands, cold feet, falling hair, and brittle fingernails. A severe deficiency of iodine results in goiter. If the thyroid gland has not been injured, the condition is corrected by an adequate diet rich in iodine.

To supply iodine, use iodized salt at all times; eat sea foods or ocean fish at least once each week.

If you live in a goiter belt, ask your physician about adding iodine to the baby's formula and to the children's food, particularly during puberty; about taking iodine during pregnancy and the menopause.

If your neck seems even slightly enlarged, ask your physician if you have an incipient goiter. In case a goiter exists, supplement your diet with iodine year after year, even after the gland has returned to normal size. Persistence in supplying sufficient iodine is tremendously important.

Vitamin D and the B complex are important in stimulating normal activity of the thyroid gland; vitamins A and C, in preventing infections of the gland.

In case of exophthalmic goiter, a diet should be unusually rich in protein, the B vitamins, vitamin A, iodine, and calcium. Since vitamin A is antagonistic to excessive thyroid hormone, physicians often recommend as much as 200,000 units daily until the pulse is normal, together with 25 milligrams or more of vitamin E to insure normal utilization of vitamin A.

24

Under no circumstances should thyroid tablets be taken except on the advice of a physician; such tablets may cause heart damage and inactivity of the thyroid gland through disuse.

YOUR MENTAL HEALTH
IS DETERMINED BY THE FOOD YOU EAT

My mind went back to certain patients I had watched who had complained of poor thinking; men and women who suffered from anemia, from a lack of iodine, and from various vitamin deficiencies; or who had failed to eat frequently enough to keep their blood sugar at a normal level.

"Walter, almost every other person who consults me about some dietary problem complains that he can't think as clearly as he used to. After a person has been embarrassed by forgetfulness many times or has paced the floor a few nights because of insomnia, he invariably broods about the possibility of going insane. There are thousands of people like that in this country. There are thousands more who are depressed, uncooperative, and grouchy simply because their diet doesn't supply enough B vitamins. I remember one woman who started taking brewers' yeast every day; whenever I saw her, she would repeat over and over, 'I haven't thought so clearly in years!' Almost every person who follows a good nutritional program for a few weeks notices a marked difference in his thinking. Plenty of children have been called dullards at school because their food didn't supply the nutrients the brain cells needed to function normally."

Every nutrient which goes to make up an adequate diet probably plays some role in maintaining mental health.

Lack of almost any one of the many B vitamins shows itself almost immediately in mental depression, tendency to worry, sluggish thinking, and pessimistic forebodings. A severe deficiency of the B vitamin, niacin, results in insanity.

Persons who fail to eat frequently have been shown to think more slowly and less clearly, and to make more frequent mistakes than persons who eat 5 or 6 times daily.

Forgetfulness, due to poor circulation to the brain, may be caused by a deficiency of iodine, thiamin, or iron.

The addition of glutamic acid to the diet of well-fed experimental animals increases their speed of learning and their ability to master more complicated problems. Glutamic acid is supplied by proteins such as meat, eggs, fish, cheese, and milk. The milk protein, lactalbumin, is 25 per cent glutamic acid. Eating cheese daily and drinking a quart of milk, buttermilk, or yogurt may pay brilliant dividends.

An adequate diet may influence morality. Dr. Price has pointed out that primitive races living on adequate diets have unusually high moral standards but that immorality becomes rampant when the same races adopt the white man's diet.

TUBERCULOSIS COULD BE CALLED
A DEFICIENCY DISEASE

As we were driving home from the hospital, Alice asked, "Do you really think TB can be prevented?"

I sighed; the old story of becoming interested in prevention long after the disease had developed.

"Well, most tuberculosis starts with colds which drag on," I began. "For years it has been possible to produce tuberculosis in animals by giving them a diet which supplies some vitamin A, although not enough. The animals' lungs become infected; they develop coughs and have lung hemorrhages. They're most susceptible to the lung disease at the age which is equivalent to the late teens and twenties of human life. Animals on identical diets except for more vitamin A have no disease, even when they're fed the organisms which cause tuberculosis. The bacteria are different from those which cause the disease in humans."

Alice was silent, and I guessed she was thinking of Pat.

"Also when two groups of animals are fed identically except for vitamin C, the deficient ones are much more susceptible when bacteria are injected directly into their lungs. I was reading recently of an experiment in which identical diets were given to seventy guinea pigs, except that half of them were given a little less orange juice than the others. All were fed tubercular bacilli by mouth; only two on the adequate diet developed tuberculosis,

26

and it was a light form, but twenty-five of the others died from the disease. Draw your own conclusions."

The light from a passing car showed that Alice's face was serious and thoughtful.

"In tuberculosis the formation of a substantial scar around the diseased part of the lung is of particular importance," I continued. "A substance in scar tissue which gives it strength—collagen—depends on vitamin C, the vitamin in oranges and grapefruit. Dr. Hojer studied this quite extensively in experimental animals with tuberculosis. If the animals were given only a little vitamin C, the scar tissue was weak and poorly formed, and the tubercular lesions weren't arrested. The animals which were given plenty of the vitamin had solid, compact scar tissue, and the disease was checked."

Tuberculosis leads all other causes of death as a killer between the ages of 15 and 35 years; its incidence is highest among the inadequately fed.

Probably all nutrients play some role in preventing tuberculosis. Experimental tuberculosis has been produced by diets undersupplied in vitamin A and by the injection of bacteria into animals deficient in vitamin C.

During active tuberculosis, the B vitamins, vitamin D, calcium, and protein should be kept more than adequate. The daily diet should supply 50,000 to 100,000 units of vitamin A and 200 to 400 milligrams of vitamin C, or ascorbic acid.

Tuberculosis is arrested when the body seals off the infected areas by a ring of calcium laid down in a bed of connective tissue. The disease becomes active again whenever calcium is so deficient that the wall cannot remain strong, when vitamin D is so undersupplied that calcium cannot be well absorbed, or when vitamin C is so lacking that the connective tissue breaks down. These nutrients must be continuously adequate if the disease is to be arrested permanently.

CAN AN ADEQUATE DIET HELP TO PREVENT CANCER?

Marie bent over a low table and flipped through the pages of a small magazine. "I read an article about the Mormons recently. It seems the founder of their religion recommended a good diet more than a hundred years ago." She picked up the magazine. "Here it is. Out of every 100,000 deaths reported in the United States and five European countries, 119 are caused by cancer. But out of every 100,000 deaths among the Latter Day Saints, only 47 are caused by cancer. A good deal less than half."

I turned, leaning my elbow on the mantel. "In isolated districts where nutrition has been found to be completely adequate, there is no cancer at all. Dr. E. H. Tipper writes in his book, *Cancer, a Disease of Civilization*, that he never found one case of cancer among some two million people of the Niger Delta, but in the African coast towns, where inadequate diets were used, cancer was rampant. Dr. Weston Price studied isolated groups of people in Switzerland, Alaska, and the South Sea Islands, and he stresses the same thing—that cancer is unknown as long as the people do not adopt the diet of civilization, which lacks vitamins and minerals. Dr. McCarrison states that during nine years of work among a group of people in the Himalayas who have magnificent physiques and whose health is far above the average, he never saw one case of cancer."

Marie leaned forward. "What do these people eat that we don't?"

"In most cases, their foods are the simple ones which any American could live on if he wanted to—milk, cheese, fruits, vegetables, glandular meats, eggs, and unmilled grains. But they aren't getting white sugar, soft drinks, cakes, pies, candies, and other refined foods which make up from a half to two-thirds of all the calories consumed by the people in our country. All the foods they eat build health; most of the foods Americans eat can only produce disease."

Outstanding researchers who have worked among primitive peoples point out that when the diet of these peoples is adequate, cancer is unknown; that when the white man's diet is adopted, cancer becomes rampant.

Cancers were induced in 96 per cent of animals given a diet mildly deficient in protein and B vitamins. When adequate amounts of milk protein and B vitamins were added to an otherwise identical diet, only 7 per cent of the animals developed cancer.

The growth of experimental tumors can be inhibited by large amounts of vitamins A and E and the B vitamins, biotin and inositol. The growth of certain types of tumors in humans has been retarded by these nutrients.

BONES CAN BE STRONG AT ANY AGE

"Poor old soul!" I hung up the receiver. "Only a few years more to live, and now she's fallen—"

"And broken her hip."

I glanced up in astonishment, amazed to realize the occurrence was so common that Betty, knowing only that I was speaking of an elderly person, could complete such a sentence.

"Saw dozens of cases when I was with Old Age Pensions. Hundreds more are worried constantly for fear they'll fall. One old lady told me she wouldn't take a tub bath any more for fear of falling and becoming crippled."

I motioned for Betty to sit down. "All experimental evidence shows that bones can be built up at any age. The medical literature is full of case histories of older people whose bones knit rapidly when given the same foods fed to children to build bones—milk, cheese, cod-liver oil, orange juice, and sufficient B vitamins to insure good absorption into the blood. However, it's easy to understand why older people's bones break easily and don't knit. Many of them have never eaten adequate amounts of calcium, never tasted cod-liver oil or taken a sunbath, certainly don't get orange juice or any other source of vitamin C every day. Unless the diet is adequate, each pregnancy and lactation period take tremendous amounts of minerals from the bones. These minerals are never put back unless the diet is more than adequate later."

When experimental animals are kept on an adequate diet, their

29

bones become progressively stronger with age. Fragile bones of elderly persons are the result of cumulative deficiencies.

The basis of bones is of protein; to maintain a strong base, generous amounts of milk, cheese, eggs, and meat must be eaten.

The elasticity of the bone base depends upon the intake of vitamin C, or ascorbic acid, which gives strength to the connective tissue; healthy bones are somewhat elastic at any age. To maintain bone health, 100 milligrams or more of this vitamin should be obtained daily.

Calcium and phosphorous give hardness to the bones; insure an adequate supply of these minerals by eating cheese daily and by drinking a quart of whole or skim milk, buttermilk, or yogurt; 1000 units or more of vitamin D must be obtained daily to insure normal utilization of these minerals.

The B vitamins, supplied by wheat germ, brewers' yeast, liver, and whole-grain breads and cereals, are necessary to insure complete absorption of calcium and phosphorus.

Broken bones heal rapidly when the daily diet includes: 80 or more grams of protein; 300 or more milligrams of vitamin C, or ascorbic acid; 3,000 units of vitamin D; and 1 to 3 grams of calcium. Tablets of a calcium salt, such as dicalcium phosphate, should be taken to supplement the food calcium until healing is complete.

ALLERGIES INDICATE THAT THE GENERAL HEALTH IS BELOW PAR

We left the building and walked across the campus.

"Allergies frequently appear after colds, bronchitis, or any condition which leaves the body run down," I said. "And it's amazing how they appear when things have gone wrong—when you're mentally upset or worried."

I knew Walter's romance with Cynthia was going none too well; that he had frequent colds and was making no effort to prevent them.

"That's the trouble with putting the entire emphasis on avoiding the foods you're allergic to," I continued. "If you're giving up milk, wheat, eggs, fish, and orange juice, chances are that you're low in protein, iron, calcium, maybe phosphorus and copper, vitamins A and C, the B vitamins, iodine, and goodness knows what else. When you don't find a substitute for the minerals, vitamins, and proteins in every valuable food which you give up, then your general health naturally suffers. The poorer your diet becomes, the more easily you get irritated, upset, depressed, and worried. It isn't much wonder the allergies get worse too, even though you may feel better temporarily by giving up the foods you're allergic to."

We found a table at the extreme end of the room, and Walter took the seat opposite me.

"My allergies don't stay the same, you know. The tests one week showed I was allergic to wheat, milk, and tomatoes; the next week I was not allergic to these at all, but to rye, fish, and orange juice. Most people assume that if they're ever allergic to a food, they're always allergic to it. I know people do get over allergies."

"They don't get over them, as a rule," I said, "unless every effort is made to build up the health."

In case of any allergy, the first and greatest emphasis should be on building health. The daily food intake should be carefully checked and made more than adequate in ever respect.

When any food must be given up temporarily, other foods which supply the same dietary factors must be substituted for that omitted. For example, if milk is avoided, 1 gram of calcium, 1.5 grams of phosphorus, 2 milligrams of vitamin B_2, or riboflavin, and 32 grams of protein should be obtained from other sources.

Excellent results have been obtained in treating allergies with large amounts of vitamin C, or ascorbic acid. Physicians often recommended that a tablet supplying 100 milligrams of this vitamin be taken every 2 or 3 hours, or as much as 600 to 800 milligrams daily. Since vitamin C is easily lost in urine, no more than 100 milligrams should be taken at one time.

Large amounts of vitamin A, or as much as 150,000 to 250,000 units taken daily for a month, appear to increase the resistance to hay fever; 25 or more milligrams of vitamin E, or alpha tocopherol, should be obtained daily to insure normal utilization of the vitamin A.

Calcium and vitamin D often decrease the severity of asthmatic attacks; 1 or 2 calcium tablets containing vitamin D may be taken each hour.

Eczemas often considered due to allergies are frequently caused by deficiencies of the lesser known B vitamins; these eczemas usually clear up when a heaping tablespoonful of brewers' yeast stirred into water is taken before each meal, between meals, and before bed for a week or more.

After following a completely adequate diet for several weeks, taste foods you have been allergic to; if no irritation results, gradually increase the amounts of these foods; if you are still allergic to them, avoid them temporarily, and repeat the procedure in a few weeks.

Many allergies are caused by the absorption of a substance known as histamine, formed by bacteria in the intestinal tract. The offending bacteria are apparently destroyed when a clove of garlic or 2 to 4 glasses of yogurt are consumed daily.

Migraine headaches, often thought of as an allergic reaction, can be produced in humans by a diet undersupplied in vitamin B_1, or thiamin. Physicians often recommend that migraine patients take 2 milligrams of thiamin every hour during headaches, and 2 milligrams with each meal when not suffering from a headache.

THE VALUE OF VITAMIN CAPSULES, TABLETS, AND CONCENTRATES

Mabel looked puzzled. "Then the vitamin capsules I'm giving the children probably don't furnish nearly all the vitamins they need."

I had been hoping that she would say just that. "No capsule can supply all the vitamins one needs; yet many people take them believing they do. Consequently, such persons eat only the foods their palates dictate instead of choosing foods which build health."

"I should think capsules would be better than nothing."

"That's true. Capsules are of tremendous value, particularly in supplying vitamin D which is not found in foods. But you have to balance the good they can do against the harm they may do. Multiple-vitamin capsules usually contain a fair amount of the cheaper vitamins. The more expensive vitamins are little more than talking points. Many of the lesser known vitamins, which may prove to be as important as the well-known ones, are usually not included at all. Yet people who might drink milk and orange juice or eat wheat germ and liver don't make any special effort to eat these foods because they think they're getting all the nutrients they need from the capsules. Health comes from eating foods which supply all the nutrients essential to promote vigor, clear thinking, freedom from illness, and a forgetfulness of the body. Vitamin capsules should be used merely as a supplement to the very best diet one can obtain."

Whenever adequate nutrition cannot be obtained from natural foods, supplement your diet with vitamin and mineral concentrates.

Synthetic, or chemically made, vitamins are identical with vitamins occurring naturally in foods, and can be taken in much larger quantities than can be obtained from food. Unrefined foods, however, supply many nutrients aside from vitamins.

Vitamins and minerals, either natural or in concentrated form, are not fattening; they contain no calories. An adequate intake of vitamins and minerals is essential to any good reducing diet.

In purchasing vitamin or mineral products, buy only those which have quantities clearly stated on the label.

Vitamin D is not supplied adequately by foods. Every person not exposed daily to ultraviolet rays from a lamp or summer sunshine should take fish-liver oil or other reliable source of vitamin D.

Capsules and tablets claiming to supply the vitamin-B complex either lack the following B vitamins or contain them in too small amounts to be significant: para aminobenzoic acid; inositol; folic acid; cholin; biotin; and others. These lesser known B vitamins may prove to be of as great importance as the well-known ones. To obtain all the B vitamins, use natural foods such as brewers' yeast, wheat germ, liver; the bacteria of yogurt, the Bulgarian cultured milk, may synthesize all the B vitamins in the intestine provided sufficient amounts are eaten.

Multi-mineral tablets are available which supply not only calcium, phosphorus, and vitamin D but also iron, copper, iodine, and the many trace minerals; when mineral supplements are required, choose these in preference to tablets supplying only calcium.

Compare the cost of the amounts of vitamins and minerals in various products before making a selection. Products which are shipped from one state to another are inspected by the Federal Food and Drug Administration and must meet the qualifications stated on the label.

Concentrates of vitamins A, D, E, and K should be taken immediately after meals; these fat-soluble vitamins are carried through the intestinal wall by substances in bile, which flows into the intestine after eating. Less of the water-soluble B vitamins and vitamin C is lost in the urine when small amounts are taken frequently than when large amounts are taken at one time.

Minerals such as calcium, phosphorus, iron and copper dissolve in acid; when mineral concentrates are used, they should be taken before meals, between meals, or before bed when there is free hydrochloric acid in the stomach. The absorption of minerals is more complete when small amounts are taken frequently than when large amounts are taken at one time.

GETTING READY FOR SURGERY

Gail was stretched out on the davenport, her eyes closed. "I dread going to the hospital. Was given a general anesthetic when I had my tonsils out. Vomiting made my throat feel awful." She groaned. "The appendix was worse still. If you want to experience the worst kind of terror, just have a fresh incision jerked and pulled by vomiting."

"Not as much was known then as now. There's little chance of your being nauseated if you eat candy, plenty of it. Any general anesthetic causes fat to be drawn into the blood stream. Besides, you may not be able to eat for a couple of days, and you'll have to live largely on fat which is stored in your body. Fats can't be burned completely without sugar. Products called ketone bodies are formed from the partially burned fat and are the cause of the nausea after an operation. However, if you eat sugar or candy just before going to the hospital, the extra fat, brought into the blood by the anesthetic, can be completely burned and the nausea prevented. Totally aside from any operation, going without eating for three or four days and living on body fat alone can cause a severe acetone acidosis—tiredness, nervousness, bad breath, headache, and nausea. Having plenty of sugar stored in your body in advance helps a great deal."

Gail gave a sigh of relief. "I'm glad to know that. How much should I eat?"

"The day before the operation, eat at least a pound. Get any kind of candy which is largely sugar. Jelly beans or marsh-mallows or gum drops are probably the best. Avoid chocolates, caramels, butterscotch, creamy bonbons, or any other food which contains fat."

These suggestions must necessarily be general and may be con-tradicted by your particular condition. Do not follow them without the permission of your physician.

Nausea following surgery can usually be prevented by having a large amount of sugar stored in your body before surgery.

Since vitamin C, or ascorbic acid, increases the speed of healing, saturate the tissues with this vitamin by obtaining 100 milli-grams with each meal, between meals, and before bed for a week prior to surgery; continue this amount of vitamin C until healing is complete. Use natural sources supplemented by ascorbic acid tablets.

To decrease gas and fermentation in the intestines, either fresh garlic or yogurt prepared with skim milk should be used liberally before surgery.

Adequate calcium and vitamins D and K aid in clotting blood

and preventing hemorrhage; mineral tablets supplying calcium should be taken 2 or 3 times daily during the week before surgery; 2,000 units or more of vitamin D should be taken daily. Vitamin K may be obtained from tablets or from green leafy vegetables.

Large amounts of body protein are destroyed following surgery; recovery is more rapid when the convalescent diet contains as much milk, eggs, cheese, and meat as can be tolerated.

PREVENTING HEART DISEASE

I happened to be going down the hall of the medical building as Pete stood in the doorway saying goodbye to his last patient. "I want to see you," he called. As I went into his office, he added, "What do you know about vitamin B and heart disease?"

"Well, functional heart disease has been produced experimentally in humans," I answered. "Dr. Russell Wilder at Mayo's produced it in girls living on a diet adequate in all respects except for vitamin B_1. Dr. Norman Jolliffe made a study of the hearts of five volunteers who lived on a similar diet. After only four days they noticed that on slight exertion they had difficulty in getting their breath. They suffered from palpitation of the heart too. Electrocardiograms showed their hearts were abnormal, and fluorscopic examination showed that the hearts were enlarged. When thiamin was given, the symptom disappeared in a few days."

"Sorry I missed reading those reports. I've no time to read half the things I want to."

"The influence of vitamin B_1 on the heart isn't new. When animals are put on a diet lacking it, the change in the heart is the first symptom to appear, according to Dr. Harris of Cambridge University. A slow pulse—bradycardia—comes even before a loss of appetite, which used to be considered the first symptom of a B_1 deficiency; the poor circulation comes long before constipation, which certainly seems to be the most common symptom of a B_1 deficiency in this country. Patients with many types of heart disease considered to be unrelated to lack of thiamin, or B_1, have been found to have abnormally small amounts of the vitamin in the blood and urine. I'd say that adequate B vitamins are more important in preventing and correcting heart disease than are any other nutrients."

Experimental heart disease has been produced in humans by placing them on a diet inadequate in thiamin, or vitamin B_1. Deaths from heart disease have increased many fold since the milling of flour has decreased the national consumption of this vitamin.

Patients with heart disease should live on a diet adequate in all respects. Approximately 6 milligrams of thiamin should be obtained daily from natural foods such as brewers' yeast, wheat germ, liver, and yogurt.

Rheumatic fever is frequently responsible for heart damage. An adequate diet particularly rich in protein and vitamin C, or ascorbic acid, helps to prevent recurring attacks of rheumatic fever, thereby protecting the heart.

Infectious heart disease appears to be secondary to infections of the tonsils, teeth, or other organs of the body. Have all dead teeth removed. Dead teeth showing no abscesses are probably more dangerous than those showing abscesses; they are more often infected by streptococcus.

FEEDING THE PERFECT BABY

I stood in the nursery looking at Betty's new baby. It's a funny thing—the way you change your mind about babies. Your first impression often is that they are quite homely; a moment later you think they're cute; and at the end of five minutes you resent it if anyone as much as insinuates they're not beautiful.

Betty, slender and attractive in a flowered housedress, came into the room carrying a bottle.

"What's that?"

"Water and vitamins."

"At three weeks? Hurrah. That's the way babies should be fed. What vitamins?"

"About three tablespoonfuls of orange juice, just to get him used to it, and a 100-milligram tablet of ascorbic acid for good measure. The water was left from steaming the potatoes and spinach last night. I salt the vegetables with iodized salt so that the baby can get his salt and iodine from the water. I shake a heaping tablespoon of brewers' yeast with the water too, and the health cocktail is ready to be served. It's no trouble at all. Instead of putting the cod-liver oil into the formula and having it stick to the bottle, I drop it directly into the baby's mouth with a large medicine dropper after each feeding.''

"You're lucky to have Dr. Williams. Many doctors don't realize how deficient a baby's diet usually is.''

I watched Betty adjust the nipple in the baby's mouth.

"Babies require a large amount of vitamin C,'' I continued. "The amount in breast milk depends entirely upon what the mother eats, and there's none in cow's milk. Iron, iodine, copper, salt, and many of the B vitamins are usually undersupplied or completely lacking from a young baby's diet. A well-fed baby is so much more fun to take care of; no constipation, vomiting, skin rashes, and that sort of thing to worry about.''

If at all possible, give the baby breast milk for at least the first few weeks. The flow of breast milk can be stimulated by a daily diet containing 3 or more tablespoons of brewers' yeast, 100 to 130 grams of protein, and 3 quarts of liquid, mostly of fruit juices and skim milk, buttermilk, or yogurt.

When the baby is two weeks old, dissolve in the formula or drinking water 100 to 300 milligrams of vitamin C, or 1 to 3 tablets of 100 milligrams each; start 1 tablespoon of orange juice and increase gradually to ½ cup daily in addition to the tablets.

To supply the B vitamins, stir 1 tablespoon of dried brewers' yeast into the baby's formula or drinking water; add yeast supplement when the baby is two weeks old; increase the amount of yeast gradually to 2 or 3 tablespoons daily by the time the baby is 6 months old; add wheat germ to all cereals or use as a cereal.

Start fish-liver oil by the end of the second week; see that 10,000 units or more of vitamin A and 2,000 units of vitamin D are supplied daily. For maximum absorption, give the oil or concentrate directly after feeding. Continue giving fish-liver oil both summer and winter until the child is grown.

For drinking water use water which vegetables have been cooked in; salt the water with iodized salt; if you live in a goiter belt, ask your pediatrician about giving a few drops of Lugol's solution.

If a formula must be given the baby, use dark or blackstrap molasses instead of the refined carbohydrates. Since blackstrap molasses is quite laxative, start by giving only 1 teaspoon, gradually increasing the amount until all refined carbohydrate is replaced.

Start all solid foods in small amounts; increase quantities gradually.

Serve cereals unsweetened; use finely ground whole-grain cereals; cook no longer than 5 or 10 minutes. Serve oatmeal, which contains phytic acid, only occasionally.

Quickly cooked vegetables prepared at home are preferrable to canned ones. Use vegetables prepared for the family; chop fine or run through food grinder.

To prevent possibility of allergies, give the baby only the yolk of hard-boiled eggs.

Start cottage cheese at 5 months and serve almost daily. Confine meats to liver, brains, spleen, and kidney, preferably quickly steamed or broiled.

Give the baby fruits for desserts. Avoid all foods made of white flour and refined sugar.

Let the baby cut his teeth on raw carrots, green peppers, celery, and similar vegetables; give red or green bell peppers daily when available.

Give the baby definite midmeals of fruit or fruit juices.

Time and effort can be saved if vegetables, fruits, and meats prepared for the baby are packed into sections of an ice tray, frozen, and reheated as needed.

Cynthia was carefully applying rouge to her cheeks. "Wish I could get my color looking decent. Nothing gives me such a dragged-out look as being without rouge."

"Nothing can give you such a dragged-out feeling as not having enough blood to produce good color either," I remarked. "The cosmetic industry is mute testimony to the value of our great American diet. Lack of color—of ears, gums, fingers, and lips, as well as cheeks—not only detracts from beauty. Any person whose coloring is poor doesn't feel as energetic or rested as he could; he can't think as clearly either. Many studies show that 90 per cent of the women and children in this country are anemic. Even a slight anemia causes unnecessary fatigue. Every time a woman puts on rouge, she should say to herself, 'I could be getting more fun out of life.' If women would do that, perhaps they'd make more attempt to obtain foods necessary to build healthy blood."

Almost every nutrient which goes to make up an adequate diet is apparently important in building blood, or in preventing and correcting anemias.

Iron is essential to give rich color to the blood; iron cannot be utilized without copper. Keep your diet adequate in these minerals by a liberal use of blackstrap molasses, liver, wheat germ, red meats, green leafy vegetables.

When calcium is undersupplied, iron combines with phosphorus and is excreted from the body; to prevent anemia, calcium and vitamin D must be adequate.

Anemias in animals can result from an undersupply of any of the following B vitamins: niacin amide, para aminobenzoic acid, folic acid, and vitamin B_6, or pyridoxin. Obtain these vitamins by the daily use of wheat germ, brewers' yeast, blackstrap molasses; eat liver 2 or more times each week.

An undersupply of iodine or vitamin C slows down the production of red blood cells in the bone marrow.

Red corpuscles are made of protein; anemia can result from a protein deficiency; it is not corrected by adding iron to the diet. When anemias are to be overcome, the protein intake should be increased 30 per cent above normal.

There is evidence that a lack of the B vitamins is a causative factor in pernicious anemia. A person suffering from this disease should supplement his daily diet with 3 or more heaping tablespoons of brewers' yeast, $\frac{1}{4}$ cup or more of wheat germ, and 1 serving of liver; at least 6 milligrams of vitamin B_1, or thiamin, should be obtained daily from natural foods.

ADEQUATE NUTRITION IS VITAL
IN TREATING ARTHRITIS

Cynthia had been telling me about her mother's arthritis.

"Does pulling teeth help arthritis?" she asked.

"Not unless the teeth are dead. They should always be removed whether they show any abscesses or not, even though the person is in perfect health. However, if a person has arthritis and an abscessed tooth, removing all infection from the mouth cannot remove the infection already in the joints."

"Have you had good results with your arthritis cases?"

I shook my head. "As a rule, the person who has arthritis is so frightened that he tries every treatment anyone recommends, from the rankest food faddist to Mayo's. Even if a certain treatment could help him, he usually doesn't stay with it long enough to get results. I suspect any one of us would be inclined to do the same."

For a moment I considered numerous patients I had seen with arthritis.

"I believe I can say that every patient who has had all known sources of infection removed, and who has followed an adequate diet day after day, has been helped. In milder cases, the mineral deposits in the joints have disappeared in 6 months; in more severe cases, it is a matter of years. Any person with arthritis should place himself in the care of a good physician who will make out an adequate diet for him, and he should eat the foods which build health day after day, year after year. If the arthritis is correctly diagnosed, and if mineral deposits are already

41

laid down in his joints, no treatment in the world can give rapid results. The patient should clearly understand that."

Experimental arthritis can be produced by injecting bacteria into animals deficient in vitamin C, or ascorbic acid; animals whose diets are adequate are not affected by the injections. Lack of vitamin C and presence of bacteria from diseased teeth or other infections are undoubtedly causative factors in human arthritis.

Excellent results have been obtained when 100 milligrams of ascorbic acid are taken in tablet form with each meal and before bed.

Citrus fruits should be largely avoided because of their high-alkaline ash; if the body fluids are allowed to become alkaline, larger amounts of minerals are deposited in the joints.

Excessive vitamin D, widely used in the treatment of arthritis, frequently results in severe toxicity: nausea, digestive upsets, insomnia, nervousness. The treatment is not sanctioned by the American Medical Association.

As in treating any infection, the protein intake should be more than adequate. Try to get at least 80 grams of protein daily, mostly from meat, fish, eggs, wheat germ, and brewers' yeast; have cheese only occasionally.

The calcium intake should be adequate (750 milligrams daily) but not excessive. This amount could best be obtained from yogurt.

Arthritis resulting from low-grade infections of the intestines usually clears when yogurt is used; have 2 or 3 glasses of yogurt daily. Fresh garlic is also recommended.

The person with arthritis should strictly avoid all concentrated sweets, soft drinks, and white flour.

A NORMAL DIGESTIVE TRACT

As soon as the new faces changed from polite boredom to flattering interest, I realized that the women were forgetting their hesitancy to stand before a group. Then I asked for their questions.

A gray-haired woman who had looked sleepy suddenly came to life. "Will the B vitamins overcome constipation if a person has taken cathartics for years?"

I nodded and smiled. "If the B vitamins are generous and the diet is adequate in other respects, the condition is usually corrected within a few days. Cathartics force the waste material through the body ahead of schedule; when they are first discontinued, there may be no waste to be evacuated for 2 or 3 days. However, cathartics and laxatives are undeniably harmful and should be discontinued. Normal elimination is stimulated by any good source of the B vitamins: wheat germ, brewers' yeast, yogurt, or liver. Blackstrap molasses is probably more laxative than any other food."

A short, overweight woman rose. "If I go a day without a bowel movement, I get a headache."

"Experiments have been carried out in which the lower part of the large intestine has been plugged with sterile cotton. About an hour later, the subjects helping with the experiment complained of headache, dizziness, bloating, and discomfort in the abdomen. Some suffered from nausea and vomiting. In other words, they developed all the symptoms of 'that poisoned feeling' we've been told for years was caused by dangerous toxins being absorbed into the blood from waste material. The symptoms completely disappeared as soon as the cotton was removed. The same thing was shown by inserting small balloons into the rectum; the more the balloons were blown up, the more severe the symtoms became. These experiments have led to the conclusion that the symptoms associated with faulty elimination are due to pressure of the hard fecal matter against delicate nerve endings."

An adequate intake of B vitamins will usually increase a poor appetite; no amount of the B vitamins will cause a normal appetite to become excessive. An excessive appetite can result from a mild deficiency of B vitamins in which sugar is not efficiently changed to energy, the blood sugar drops below normal, and a craving for sweets results.

Foods do not ferment in the normal stomach. "Burps" indicate that the person has wolfed his food and/or gulped liquids, thereby swallowing excessive amounts of air. Such difficulty can be overcome by eating slowly, chewing all food thoroughly, and sipping all liquids.

The fact that foods such as onions, garlic, or green peppers "repeat" does not indicate that these foods cause indigestion but only that aromatic oils have passed into an air bubble in the stomach; as the air bubble escapes, the flavor of the food is brought back into the mouth.

Gas, indigestion, and flatulence in the intestinal tract can usually be overcome by eating fresh garlic or by drinking 2 or more cups of yogurt daily, either of which helps to kill unfavorable bacteria in the intestines.

"Strong-flavored" vegetables, as onions, cabbage, cauliflower, Brussels sprouts, form gas only when overcooked. Cook these vegetables no longer than 8 to 10 minutes in as little water as possible; serve them while still slightly crisp.

Faulty elimination results from deficiencies of the B vitamins. It may be overcome by the daily use of 2 tablespoons or more each of brewers' yeast and blackstrap molasses, ¼ cup or more of wheat germ.

Diarrhea or the tendency to diarrhea may result from infections of the intestinal tract, from emotional upsets or from lack of niacin amide. Physicians frequently recommend 50 milligrams of niacin amide at each meal until elimination is normal. The daily use of garlic and yogurt is indicated if bacterial infection is suspected. If emotional upsets appear to be the case, consult a psychiatrist.

No food is "hard to digest." Some foods digest more rapidly and/or more completely than others. Some people have more efficient digestion and absorption of foods than others.

TIPS ON VIRILITY

There was a great deal of whispering at the other end of the table, and Jerry stood up. "The men want me to ask you if diet has any effect upon virility."

"Apparently there's a definite relation between the two. Dr. McLester states that during World War I when the nutrition was poor, men reported decreased sex interest. Animals on poor diets, particularly diets inadequate in vitamins A and E and the B vitamins, will not mate even with normal animals. The B vitamins have been found to stimulate normal glandular activity, and this includes the sex glands as well as others. Vitamin E is believed to have direct effect upon the reproductive organs, but apparently it has little to do with libido unless this vitamin is completely deficient from the diet. A lack of vitamin E in the diets of male animals causes a permanent sterility which cannot be overcome later by eating large amounts of the vitamin. If sex interest is already normal, improved nutrition, of course, will not increase it above normal. However, it has been reported clinically that sex interest has increased after a good nutrition program has taken the place of a poor one."

Normal virility is a result of general good health; all nutrients which go to make up an adequate diet play some part, directly or indirectly, in maintaining such virility.

Protein deficiency quickly results in lack of libido, or sex desire. Partial sterility in men is caused by a lack of the amino acid, arginine, which is normally supplied by the complete proteins, eggs, milk, cheese, and meats.

To promote normal virility, use generous amounts of foods rich in the B vitamins: wheat germ, brewers' yeast, blackstrap molasses, liver, whole-grain breads and cereals.

Lack of iodine in women results in lowered libido; keep iodine intake adequate by continuous use of iodized salt; if you live in a goiter belt, ask your physician about supplementing your diet with kelp or other forms of iodine.

Vitamin E, or alpha tocopherol, although known as the anti-sterility vitamin, does not appear to increase libido; this vitamin is required for the normal production of spermatozoa in males and for the normal completion of pregnancy in females.

The Bulgarians are noted for their virility extending into late life; this virility is said to be due to their daily use of yogurt, possibly because of the protein and the probable synthesis of B vitamins by the yogurt bacteria in the intestine.

When conception is desired, the diet of both the prospective mother and father should be adequate in every respect; inability to conceive can result from lack of protein, the B vitamins, or iodine.

SOUND SLEEP WITHOUT DRUGS

Cynthia leaned against the door casing, a look of distress on her face. "Dad has so much trouble sleeping; gets up and prowls around the house at three and four o'clock in the morning."

"Insomnia can easily be corrected by adequate nutrition," I answered. "I try to get my patients to drink 4 glasses of milk, buttermilk, or yogurt daily, have cheese twice daily, and take 2 cod-liver-oil capsules each day until they're sleeping better. If that doesn't bring results, I have them eat calcium tablets. Taking calcium before bed usually makes a person sleep like a kitten. One of my patients even calls his calcium tablets his lullaby pills. If everyone who takes sleeping tablets would take calcium instead, the national health record could really be improved."

Use of sleeping tablets causes tension of nerve and muscle tissue. As a result, it becomes progressively more difficult for a person to have sound sleep without drugs. The use of such tablets does untold harm.

Of all nutrients, adequate calcium is probably most important in inducing sound sleep. If you have difficulty in getting to sleep, drink a quart of milk daily and have 1 or more servings of cheese. See that you receive 1500 to 2000 units of vitamin D to insure adequate absorption of calcium.

When insomnia is a problem, obtain mineral tablets containing calcium; take 2 or 3 tablets before going to bed; keep tablets by the bedside, and if wakeful during the night, take 2 or 3 more tablets.

Vitamin B_6, or pyridoxin, appears to have a strongly sedative effect. Obtain this vitamin from wheat germ, brewers' yeast, blackstrap molasses, liver. Take a heaping tablespoon of yeast during the evening; if wakeful, sip yeast during the night.

KEEP YOUR SKIN BEAUTIFUL

Mabel rolled over on her stomach and dug her toes into the clean sand. "A lack of any one of a dozen vitamins causes an eczema, or a dermatitis." She looked up at me. "Right?"

"At least in animals. I've never seen a case of eczema which didn't clear up after getting large amounts of the B vitamins from natural sources."

"When there's a lack of vitamin A, the skin changes much the same as the mucous membranes do, doesn't it?" Mabel asked. "Grows faster than normally, but cells die and slough off all the time?"

I nodded. "The contents of whiteheads and blackheads have been found to be almost entirely dead cells, together with some oil. The cells which die and slough off in the under layers of skin do the harm. If bacteria get to them and start multiplying, then there's a boil or a pimple—pus, white blood cells, mucus. If the under layers of skin can be kept so healthy that there are no dead cells for bacteria to live on, there's little danger of acne and boils."

A completely adequate diet is necessary to insure the health of the skin; particular attention should be paid to nutrients which help to maintain normal circulation, such as iodine and thiamin, or vitamin B_1.

A lack of vitamin A results in rough skin, caused by pores being plugged with dead cells; the rough condition is most often found on the upper arms, thighs, and buttocks; pimples, boils, and carbuncles occur when these dead cells become infected.

Infections of the skin, such as impetigo, pimples, boils, and carbuncles, have been successfully treated with 150,000 units of vitamin A daily. Since vitamin E, or alpha tocopherol, is necessary before vitamin A is efficiently utilized, 10 to 20 milligrams of this vitamin daily usually speeds recovery. To accelerate healing and to increase resistance to further infections, at least 100 milligrams of vitamin C, or ascorbic acid, should be obtained with each meal. When the infection is severe, 100-milligram tablets of ascorbic acid should be taken every 3 hours.

Lack of vitamin B_2, or riboflavin, often results in a greasy or oily skin; if the deficiency is severe, a condition known as acne rosacea often occurs. Acne rosacea may also result from faulty absorption of riboflavin even when sufficient amounts are obtained in the diet.

Eczemas of many varieties may result from deficiencies of any of the following B vitamins: riboflavin, or vitamin B_2; niacin amide; vitamin B_6, or pyridoxin; biotin; para aminobenzoic acid; and possibly folic acid, inositol, and pantothenic acid. Severe eczemas have been treated successfully by 6 heaping tablespoons of brewers' yeast daily.

When skin abnormalities are the result of allergies, an intake of 100 milligrams of vitamin C, or ascorbic acid, every 3 hours, taken in the form of tablets, has produced the best results.

NEURITIS CAN BE PREVENTED

After dinner I lay in a handwoven Mexican hammock, and Pete sat beside me in a comfortable deck chair.

"I've been getting excellent results with my neuritis cases," he began. "Whenever I've given very large amounts of vitamin B_1, the patients have felt better the first week."

The pines smelled so good that I inhaled deeply before answering. "Dr. Borsook has been studying trifacial neuralgia, which is more difficult to clear up than other types of neuritis. He's been giving intravenous injections of B_1—thiamin chloride —together with foods rich in all the B vitamins. All of his patients had marked relief within 3 to 4 weeks, but they weren't entirely free from pain for months. About the time you think it's cured, it has a habit of sneaking back again, although not as severe, of course. Incidentally, he could not obtain satisfactory results by injections of thiamin alone. All the B vitamins apparently work together. To get the best results, all of them must be supplied, and they can be obtained only from food."

Neuritis, or pain following the nerve channels, is often spoken of as rheumatism; neuralgia; lumbago, or neuritis of the lumbar region of the back; sciatica, or neuritis of the sciatic nerve;

trifacial neuralgia, or neuritis of the nerves to the face; and shingles, or neuritis of the nerve endings.

Since all the B vitamins appear to work together, injections of thiamin alone have not given satisfactory results in treating neuritis.

Neuritis often indicates that an infection exists in the body and that bacteria are stealing the available supply of thiamin. Dead teeth, particularly those which show no abscesses, are frequently the offenders; in such cases, the neuritis clears up as soon as the teeth are removed and the diet is made adequate.

Chronic alcohol users are particularly subject to neuritis, both because their intake of foods rich in B vitamins is low and because alcohol increases the requirement for these vitamins. Alcoholic neuritis can be corrected by generous amounts of thiamin together with the entire B complex.

Any person who suffers from neuritis should obtain 6 to 8 milligrams of thiamin daily from natural foods. Until the pain disappears, 3-milligram tablets of thiamin should be taken approximately every 2 hours. The tablets should be discontinued as soon as the symptoms have cleared; the natural food sources should be continued indefinitely.

YOUR CHOICE OF FOODS
DETERMINES YOUR DENTAL HEALTH

Dr. Donald Sherwood kept one hand in my mouth and picked up another instrument. "Bacteria are in all mouths, whether there's decay or not. Every dentist has seen mouths which were filthy and yet free from decay. The people with the best teeth— primitive races—never heard of a toothbrush. These facts show that the tooth itself must become susceptible to decay."

I nodded.

"It's my opinion that all pyorrhea could be arrested and the bone saved if we could get the patient interested early enough," Don continued. "If two-thirds of the bone around the teeth—the alveolar process—is lost, then about all one can do is to remove the teeth. I put it squarely up to the patient: he must stay on an adequate diet, or he will probably lose his teeth. I tell him that

I can remove the infection, but I can't prevent the gums from being reinfected and I can't build up the bone. The same is true with decay. It's up to each patient to save his own teeth. All I can do is to help."

The principal cause of decay appears to be the eating of concentrated sweets such as candy, soft drinks, jams, jellies, honey, refined molasses, and desserts. If your teeth are susceptible to decay, avoid these foods as much as possible.

Probably every nutrient which goes to make up an adequate diet helps in one way or another to prevent tooth decay. The diet should be especially adequate in vitamins C and D, the B vitamins, calcium, and phosphorus. Midmeals of fruits and milk should be eaten to prevent a craving for sweets.

Pyorrhea is primarily due to a subtle but long-standing deficiency of vitamin C. The disease may be arrested by a completely adequate diet rich in calcium, vitamins A, C, D, and the B complex.

Erosion is usually caused by deficiencies of calcium and vitamin D, by faulty absorption of these nutrients, by an intake of excessive amounts of vitamin D or thyroid, or by too much sweets and refined foods. If an adequate diet is followed, erosion can be arrested.

Vincent's disease, or trench mouth, appears to occur only when a deficiency of the B vitamin, niacin amide, exists. Studies have shown that 150 milligrams of this vitamin daily corrects the condition more quickly than do other treatments. Healing is also speeded up by generous intake of vitamins C and A.

Formation of tartar, or calculus, appears to be more rapid when vitamin A is undersupplied.

Fish-liver oil, citrus juices, milk, and cheese should be increased in the diet before and after extractions. As much as 400 milligrams of vitamin C daily is often recommended in order to accelerate healing. To prevent danger of hemorrhage, calcium tablets should be taken several days prior to extractions.

Loss of bone surrounding the teeth may indicate lack of calcium, phosphorus, protein, the B vitamins, or vitamins D or C. Experimental studies have shown that when the diet is adequate, bone surrounding the teeth becomes stronger with age.

I stood in the doorway, thinking that the furnishings of the room were so like Cynthia's parents: old and dreary, yet genuine and good; the solid mahogany and walnut, the hearts of the two kindly Middle Westerners. Cynthia's parents were old at sixty, but they had expected to be and were as resigned to it as the tables and chairs seemed to be of their scars and loss of sheen.

"Wish I could go," Cynthia said longingly. "Have to stay home and cook for the folks. No matter how completely I get the meal ready to cook, mother will leave it in the refrigerator. 'We weren't very hungry,' she always says. 'Only wanted a little toast with jam and tea.' They try to economize on food while I try to figure out how to pay the doctor bills."

"I know. People like your parents don't believe in nutrition. Even if they did, they'd think they were too old for it to do any good."

"What can I do? Tea, crackers, white bread, a little soup, an occasional egg, and sometimes microscopic servings of vegetables. Of course they don't take much exercise."

I shook my head. "That's all the more reason they should choose their foods carefully. The more a person eats, the more vitamins and minerals he gets without worrying about it. The reverse is equally true."

Since the food habits of elderly persons are usually faulty and their food intake is small, their diets are notoriously deficient in almost every respect.

A lack of vitamin C and of protein appears to be a causative factor in arterial sclerosis; satisfactory results have been obtained in treating this type of sclerosis with an adequate diet rich in these two nutrients.

In case of high blood pressure, every effort should be made to keep the diet adequate. Calcium, vitamin D, and the entire B complex are necessary to afford maximum relaxation; 300 milligrams of vitamin C should be obtained daily to prevent the walls of the blood vessels from breaking readily under the abnormal pressure. The protein intake should not be reduced. Small frequent meals, or 3 small meals and 3 large midmeals, should be eaten. Excellent results in reducing high blood pressure have been obtained by giving 150,000 units of vitamin A daily for 2 or more weeks, together with vitamin E which is needed before vitamin A can be well utilized. Emotional upsets, vigorous exercise, overeating, and the use of stimulants should be avoided.

In planning a diet for elderly persons, particular attention should be given to foods which promote normal vision (see page 15).

Vitamin and mineral concentrates, capsules, and tablets should be relied upon whenever an adequate diet cannot be obtained from natural foods.

Prostatitis and kidney and bladder infections indicate a need for generous amounts of vitamins A, C, and the B vitamins. The urine should be kept acid by the use of ½ cup or more of wheat germ daily, 1 serving of meat, 1 egg, and a limited use of citrus fruits. Vitamin C, or ascorbic acid, should be obtained from tablets. The coli bacteria can be decreased by eating fresh garlic and/or 2 or more cups of yogurt daily.

When only a small amount of food can be eaten, the intake should be restricted largely to dairy products, glandular meats, citrus juices, wheat germ, brewers' yeast, and green and yellow fruits and vegetables. The daily use of yogurt is probably more important than that of any other one food.

ADEQUATE NUTRITION BUILDS THE BODY AS A WHOLE

Very few patients had come to the clinic that morning. When I went to the clubroom to get my coat, I found Pete and Don talking diet in front of the open fire.

Pete smiled as I joined them. "You say nutrition boils down to the simple foods we feed babies." He turned back to Don. "I'm afraid I agree with you. It's a tremendous subject. More important than I realized before I really started to study it."

"That's right," Don agreed. "An adequate diet, like sufficient sleep, excercise, fresh air, and sunshine, must come first if disease is to be prevented."

Pete leaned against the mantel. "Nutrition's only one factor. We have to remember all the influences summed up as environment and heredity."

"Of course," I agreed. "I think the best explanation of the role of nutrition in the prevention of disease throughout the entire body is McCarrison's* progression from health to disease. Do you know that?"

Pete shook his head.

I took a long breath. "First comes *faulty food*. In other words, our only standard has been taste. Then *faulty nutrition*. The minerals, sugar, vitamins, and other body needs aren't supplied, they are lacking in the tissue fluids, and the cells all over the body suffer, even though one group may suffer more than others and lead one to think that they alone are harmed. Next is *faulty function*. The eyes without vitamin A can't see well; the heart without vitamin B_1 slows down; the capillaries without vitamin C break and perhaps spill bacteria into the tissues, and so on. As a result, *faulty structure*. The muscles of the heart lose tone and may become waterlogged when B_1 isn't supplied. The bones and teeth deprived of minerals become porous; healthy compact layers of cells give place to cheesy masses of decay when vitamin A is inadequate. Then comes *faulty health*. Dangerous organisms have found their way to the dead cells. The heart muscles are too weak, or perhaps too irritated, to contract normally; circulation becomes abnormal; sufficient food and air cannot reach the tissues, and not all the wastes can be removed. So at last comes *disease*, and perhaps death."

We were silent a moment, gazing at the glowing logs.

"Of course I picked out specific examples," I continued, "but you can't recommend a nutrition program which will build up one part of the body without having it affect the entire body."

Don stood thinking, his eyes closed. "Let's see if I can quote something Socrates said about that. Memorized it once." He spoke slowly at first, gathering momentum later. "I dare say you have heard eminent physicians tell a patient who comes to them with bad eyes, that they cannot treat the eyes by themselves, but that if the eyes are to be cured, the head must be

McCarrison, Robert, Nutrition in Health and Disease. Brit. M. J., 2, 611, 1936.

treated. And then again they say that to think of the head alone, and not of the rest of the body also, is the highest of folly. And arguing thus, they apply their methods to the whole body, and try to treat and heal the whole and part together." He smiled a little bitterly. "Twenty-five hundred years ago, they poisoned the guy who knew that much."

Pete smiled. "Your quotation reminded me of one from First Corinthians." He paused for a moment. "'God framed the body on principles of compensations, by giving additional dignity to whatever part showed any deficiency, so as to prevent anything like disunion in the body, and to secure in all organs alike the same anxious care for one another's welfare. And accordingly, if one of them is in pain, all the rest are in pain with it; and honor done to one is a joy to all.'"

After a long silence we put on our coats. I kept repeating to myself, "Honor done to one is a joy to all." No one was in the mood for talking after that.

APPENDIX

LIMITATIONS OF ANY TABLE OF FOOD ANALYSIS

Many physicians and nutritionists have criticized the use of tables of food analysis, some even arguing that such tables should not be published. The principal reason is that the nutrients in foods vary widely, depending upon numerous factors: the season in which the foods were grown; the amount of sunshine, rainfall, or water they received; the degree of ripeness or maturity when harvested; the method of fertilizing the soil; and particularly upon the amount of valuable bacteria, fungi, and humus in the soil and the minerals in the topsoil and subsoil. Thus potatoes or bunches of spinach grown in various localities have different nutritive values. Carrots, for example, have been analyzed which contain no vitamin A (carotene) whatsoever. The protein content of wheat, hence of breads and cereals, can vary from 3 to 22 per cent, depending upon the humus content of the soil. The nutritive value of milk, eggs, and meats vary with the diet of the animals which produced them. The losses which occur during harvesting, shipping, storing, processing, marketing, and preparing and cooking foods at home cause the nutritive values to vary much more. Although the analyses of foods in the following table were made at many universities and by reputable laboratories and are correct for the specific samples of food used, the foods you actually serve your family may have a far different analysis.

Another criticism is that such tables leave the impression that the nutrients listed are more important than those omitted: vitamins D, E, K, and P, and many B vitamins, and numerous minerals. One or more of these nutrients may be particularly vital to your individual health. Furthermore, even when a food is known to contain a certain nutrient, there is no assurance that it will be efficiently absorbed into your blood or not destroyed in the body or lost in the excreta.

The following table, however, may be used as a general guide in planning your menus provided you appreciate its limitations.

APPENDIX

Weights:

1 gamma, or microgram	= one-millionth of a gram
1000 gammas, or micrograms	= 1 milligram
1000 milligrams	= 1 gram
28.35 grams	= 1 ounce

Abbreviations:

International unit is abbreviated as **I.U.**

United States Pharmacopeia unit, is abbreviated **U.S.P.** unit.

Relation of weights to units:

1 milligram thiamin	= 333 I.U., or U.S.P. units
1 milligram riboflavin	= 333 Sherman-Bourquin units
1 milligram ascorbic acid	= 20 I.U., or U.S.P. units
1 I.U., or U.S.P. unit, of vitamin A	= 0.6 gamma of beta-carotene
1 I.U., or U.S.P. unit, of thiamin	= 3 gammas of thiamin chloride
1 I.U., or U.S.P. unit, of ascorbic acid	= 0.05 milligrams of ascorbic acid
1 I.U., or U.S.P. unit, of vitamin D	= 0.025 gammas of vitamin D_2
1 Sherman-Bourquin unit of riboflavin	= 3 gammas of riboflavin

Conversion tables:

To convert milligrams of calcium and phosphorus to grams, divide by 1000 by moving the decimal point three places to the left.

To convert gammas of thiamin and riboflavin to milligrams, divide by 1000 by moving the decimal point three places to the left.

To convert I.U., or U.S.P. units, of thiamin or riboflavin to gammas, multiply by 3.

To convert I.U., or U.S.P. units, of ascorbic acid to milligrams, divide by 20.

*Pages in this appendix are due to the courtesy of The Macmillian Company, publishers of Vitality Through Planned Nutrition, by Adelle Davis in which these pages originally appeared substantially in their present form.

In the following table, in order to avoid decimals, amounts of calcium and phosphorus are given in milligrams instead of grams, and thiamin and riboflavin in gammas rather than milligrams. Vitamins A and D are in International, or United States Pharmacopeia units; ascorbic acid is in milligrams. With the exception of milk, average servings of food are given; weights and measures are of edible portions only. In case of cereals and legumes, raw weights are given with approximate cooked measure. Figures are for pasteurized milk and sulphur-dried fruits. Unless specified, vitamin and mineral contents are for uncooked foods, and allowances must be made for losses during cooking.

FOOD	WEIGHT, GRAMS	MEASURE	VITAMINS A UNITS	THIAMIN GAMMAS
almonds	10	10 med.	0	15
apple	100	1 sm.	90	36
applesauce, sweetened	100	½ c.	60	25
apricots, dried	50	8 halves	6850	48
apricots, fresh	100	6 halves	7500	33
artichoke, Jerusalem	50	1 med.	200	75
asparagus, bleached	100	8 st.	0	150
asparagus, green	100	8 st.	1100	360
avocado	100	½ med.	500	120
bacon, crisp	10	1½ sl.	0	27
banana	100	1 med.	300	45
barley, pearl	100	½ c. raw	0	165
barley, whole	100	½ c. raw	—	2200
beans, kidney, cooked	100	½ c.	300	216
beans, Lima, dry, cooked	90	½ c.	0	300

ABBREVIATIONS USED IN TABLE

* *probably rich source*	oz. *ounce*	sq. *square*
— *amount insignificant*	in. *inch*	sm. *small*
.. *no data available*	lg. *large*	st. *stalk*
av. *average*	med. *medium*	T. *tablespoonful*
c. *standard measuring cup*	ser. *serving*	t. *teaspoonful*
	sl. *slice*	

EQUIVALENT MEASURES OF QUANTITY

3 t. = 1 tablespoonful
16 T. = 1 standard measuring cup
8 oz. = 1 cup
32 oz. = 1 quart

VITAMINS			CALCIUM MILLIGRAMS	PHOSPHORUS MILLIGRAMS	IRON MILLIGRAMS	PROTEIN GRAMS	CALORIES
RIBOFLAVIN GAMMAS	ASCORBIC ACID MILLIGRAMS	D UNITS					
10	1	0	25	45	0.3	2	65
50	6	0	7	12	0.3	0	64
75	5	0	10	18	0.4	0	150
250	0	0	16	30	0.8	1	102
100	4	0	13	24	0.6	1	70
15	10	0	20	47	0.4	1	32
65	12	0	21	40	1	2	20
65	20	0	21	40	1	2	20
137	9	0	44	42	6.3	2	263
7	0	0	0	3	0.1	2	53
87	10	0	8	28	0.6	1	85
0	0	0	20	181	0.2	38	330
..	0	0	51	400	4.7	36	310
210	0	0	46	152	0.6	6	88
250	0	0	72	386	2.9	8	129

FOOD	WEIGHT, GRAMS	MEASURE	VITAMINS A UNITS	VITAMINS THIAMIN GAMMAS
beans, Lima, green, cooked	100	½ c.	900	225
beans, navy, baked	100	½ c.	20	150
beans, string, green, cooked	100	¾ c.	950	60
beef broth	200	1 c.	0	..
beef, fat	113	4 oz. or 1 sl.	40	135
beef, lean	113	4 oz. or 1 sl.	60	140
beet greens, cooked	135	½ c.	22,000	100
beets	100	½ c.	50	41
blackberries	100	¾ c.	300	25
blueberries	100	¾ c.	35	45
bologna	50	10 sl. sm.	0	255
brains, beef	113	4 oz.	54	168
bran, wheat flakes	25	1 c.	25	240
bread, rye	30	1 sl.	—	66
bread, white, milk	30	1 sl.	10	15
bread, white, roll	50	1 lg.	12	24
bread, wholewheat, 100%	30	1 sl.	10	180
broccoli, flower	100	¾ c.	6000	120
broccoli, leaf	100	¾ c.	30,000	120
broccoli, stem	100	¾ c.	2000	..
Brussels sprouts	100	¾ c.	400	180
buckwheat, whole	100	5 T.	..	660
butter	10	2 t., 1 sq.	225	12
buttermilk	960	1 qt.	400	300
cabbage, inside leaves	100	1 c. raw	0	78

VITAMINS			CALCIUM MILLI-GRAMS	PHOSPHO-RUS MILLI-GRAMS	IRON MILLI-GRAMS	PROTEIN GRAMS	CALORIES
RIBOFLAVIN GAMMAS	ASCORBIC ACID MIL-LIGRAMS	D UNITS					
250	42	0	21	130	0.9	7	116
15	0	0	52	155	3.8	6	115
100	8	0	55	50	1.1	2	43
..	0	0	0	..	..	4	30
200	0	0	12	204	3	19	242
262	0	0	13	214	3.4	22	190
500	50	0	94	40	3.2	2	28
37	8	0	28	42	2.8	2	40
30	3	0	32	32	0.9	0	52
31	11	0	25	20	0.9	0	50
200	0	0	40	102	4.2	8	109
360	18	..	16	340	5.3	11	127
80	0	0	30	305	1.9	1	70
..	0	0	12	74	0.6	3	76
20	0	0	14	32	0.2	3	72
25	0	0	12	40	0.2	4	100
100	0	0	22	102	1.1	3	75
350	65	0	64	105	1.3	2	35
687	90	0	262	67	2.3	3	35
187	..	0	83	35	1.1	2	35
90	130	0	27	121	2.1	4	55
..	0	0	24	306	2.6	12	240
0	0	4	1	1	0	0	77
1850	0	5	1200	960	—	30	400
75	50	0	46	34	0.2	2	28

FOOD	WEIGHT, GRAMS	MEASURE	VITAMINS	
			A UNITS	THIAMIN GAMMAS
cabbage, Chinese	100	1 c. raw	5000	36
cabbage, green	100	1 c. raw	160	90
cake, chocolate	50	1 sl.	160	15
cake, devil's food	50	1 sl.	150	19
cake, sponge	25	1 sl.	160	36
candy, chocolate	15	1 piece	—	0
candy, chocolate nut	40	1 bar	—	..
candy, gumdrop	10	1 lg.	0	0
candy, marshmallow	6	1 av.	0	0
candy, milk chocolate	50	1 bar	—	0
candy, mint	6	1 piece	—	0
candy, peanut brittle	25	2x3x¼ in.	0	45
cantaloupe (see melon)				
carrots	100	½ c. diced	4500	70
cashew nuts	30	20 nuts	0	*
cauliflower	100	¾ c.	10	85
celery, bleached	100	4 st.	20	30
celery, green	100	4 st.	640	30
celery root	100	½ c.	..	..
cereal, whole wheat, cooked	100	⅔ c.	7	140
chard, leaves, cooked	100	½ c.	15,000	450
cheese, American	40	2x1x1 in.	1000	18
cheese, Cheddar	30	2 T.	500	45
cheese, cottage	100	½ c.	180	18
cheese, cream	20	1 T.	3500	10
cheese, Swiss	30	1 sl.	660	..

VITAMINS			CALCIUM MILLI-GRAMS	PHOSPHO-RUS MILLI-GRAMS	IRON MILLI-GRAMS	PROTEIN GRAMS	CALORIES
RIBOFLAVIN GAMMAS	ASCORBIC ACID MIL-LIGRAMS	D UNITS					
462	50	0	400	72	2.5	2	30
150	50	0	429	72	2.8	2	28
30	0	0	21	48	0.4	3	200
37	0	0	11	101	2.9	3	177
6	0	..	18	55	0.8	2	72
0	0	0	0	0	0	—	45
..	0	0	0	—	0	5	219
0	0	0	0	0	0	1	36
0	0	0	0	0	0	—	20
0	0	0	10	—	0	4	282
0	0	0	0	0	0	0	20
30	0	0	5	26	0.4	3	115
75	5	0	45	41	0.6	1	30
76	0	0	16	160	..	6	202
90	75	0	122	60	0.9	2	25
15	5	0	78	46	0.5	1	19
45	7	0	98	46	0.8	1	19
..	2	0	47	71	0.8	3	38
30	0	0	10	98	1.4	3	100
165	37	0	150	50	3.1	2	25
200	0	0	380	274	0.4	12	160
650	0	0	254	181	0.1	7	100
250	0	—	995	374	—	19	100
112	0	—	127	104	—	2	75
150	0	—	330	281	0.4	10	135

FOOD	WEIGHT, GRAMS	MEASURE	VITAMINS A UNITS	THIAMIN GAMMAS
cherries, stoned	100	12 lg.	259	51
chestnuts, fresh	20	6 nuts	0	48
chicken	113	4 oz.	0	140
chocolate malted milk	350	13 oz.	2260	333
chocolate milk shake	350	13 oz.	1240	168
chocolate pudding [1]	125	½ c.	592	15
chocolate, sweetened	30	1 oz.	0	25
clams	113	6, or ¾ c.	20	21
coca cola	200	7 oz.	0	0
cocoa [2]	150	1 c.	300	30
cocoanut, dried	20	3 T.	..	15
cod-liver oil, U.S.P.	15	1 T.	10,000	0
cod fish	113	4 oz.	10	150
coffee, liquid	200	1 c.	0	0
collards, cooked	100	½ c.	6300	130
cookie, molasses	25	1 lg.	—	—
corn, canned, yellow	100	½ c.	900	130
corn, on cob, yellow	100	1 med.	860	209
corn oil	11	1 T.	0	0
corned beef	113	4 oz.	..	..
cornflakes	20	¾ c.	0	20
cornmeal, white	100	½ c.	0	110
cornmeal, yellow	100	½ c.	500	110
cottonseed oil	11	1 T.	0	0
crab	113	⅔ c.	..	135
Crackers, graham	20	2	0	48

[1] 100 gm. milk, ¼ egg
[2] 100 gm. milk

VITAMINS			CALCIUM MILLI-GRAMS	PHOSPHO-RUS MILLI-GRAMS	IRON MILLI-GRAMS	PROTEIN GRAMS	CALORIES
RIBOFLAVIN GAMMAS	ASCORBIC ACID MIL-LIGRAMS	D UNITS					
—	12	0	19	30	0.4	1	90
..	0	0	7	19	0.8	—	37
180	0	0	14	232	3.1	18	125
532	0	10	390	306	1.1	11	514
432	0	10	390	300	0.9	10	472
150	0	4	149	164	—	5	272
..	0	0	27	130	0.7	—	170
15	15	5	95	93	4.2	14	100
0	0	0	0	0	0	0	135
150	0	1	186	62	0.4	5	135
25	0	0	12	31	0.4	1	130
0	0	1700	0	0	0	0	100
192	0	—	12	120	0.6	16	70
0	0	0	0	0	0	0	0
*	70	0	207	75	3.4	3	41
..	0	0	39	25	1.5	2	100
120	4	0	6	103	0.4	4	120
55	8	0	8	103	0.4	3	90
0	0	0	0	0	0	0	100
*	0	0	13	119	6.8	16	196
20	0	0	10	38	0.1	2	100
82	0	0	16	152	0.5	8	270
100	0	0	16	152	0.9	8	272
0	0	0	0	0	0	0	100
420	12	..	17	181	0.1	16	80
..	0	0	4	20	0.2	2	84

FOOD	WEIGHT, GRAMS	MEASURE	VITAMINS	
			A UNITS	THIAMIN GAMMAS
crackers, soda	12	2 lg.	0	0
cranberries, sauce	100	¾ c.	30	0
cream, table, 20%	60	4 T.	510	30
cream, whipping, 40%	60	4 T.	1020	30
cream soup, spinach [1]	150	¾ c.	4800	87
cream soup, tomato [1]	150	¾ c.	1100	96
cucumbers	100	1 med.	35	60
custard [2]	130	½ c.	918	48
dandelion greens, cooked	100	½ c.	20,000	190
dates, dried, stoned	100	15 med.	155	60
doughnuts	100	2	190	18
duck	113	4 oz.	..	360
egg, whole	50	1 av.	600	65
egg white	30	1 white	0	5
egg yolk	20	1 yolk	600	60
eggplant	100	½ c.	70	42
endive	100	10 st.	15,000	58
escarol (chicory)	100	¾ c.	23,000	75
farina, raw, refined	20	3 T.	0	10
figs, dried	30	2 sm.	15	15
figs, fresh	50	2 lg.	50	37
fish (average)	113	4 oz.	16	148
flour, buckwheat	113	1 c.	0	300
flour, rye	113	1 c.	0	171
flour, soy bean	113	1 c.	..	650

[1] ½ c. milk, whole
3 T. vegetable

[2] ½ c. milk, whole
½ egg

VITAMINS			CALCIUM MILLIGRAMS	PHOSPHORUS MILLIGRAMS	IRON MILLIGRAMS	PROTEIN GRAMS	CALORIES
RIBOFLAVIN GAMMAS	ASCORBIC ACID MILLIGRAMS	D UNITS					
0	0	0	2	10	0	1	53
0	6	0	13	11	0.4	—	300
90	0	5	45	40	—	2	105
90	0	10	38	36	—	1	240
150	2	4	157	144	3.5	5	150
150	3	4	130	140	0.6	4	141
54	12	0	10	21	0.3	1	15
225	0	6	134	175	0.7	7	126
270	100	0	84	35	6	3	45
54	0	0	70	56	3.5	2	347
87	0	0	21	55	1.6	7	481
..	0	0	10	200	2.3	21	159
150	0	50	32	112	1.5	6	75
50	0	0	4	5	0	3	12
100	0	50	28	107	1.5	3	58
36	10	0	11	31	0.5	1	15
72	20	0	104	39	1.2	1	8
250	7	0	29	27	1.5	1	20
0	0	0	5	25	0.1	2	72
32	0	0	54	38	0.7	1	103
30	1	0	26	18	0.4	1	42
220	0	..	12	128	1.6	21	140
..	0	0	11	193	1.3	6	387
72	0	0	18	289	1.4	9	388
370	0	0	200	450	7.4	37	379

FOOD	WEIGHT, GRAMS	MEASURE	VITAMINS	
			A UNITS	THIAMIN GAMMAS
flour, wheat, fortified[1]	113	1 c.	0	450
flour, wheat, refined	113	1 c.	0	70
flour, wheat, whole grain	113	1 c.	42	450
frankfurters	113	2 links	0	*
gelatin, dried	10	1 T.	0	0
gingerale	200	7 oz.	0	0
goose	113	4 oz.	..	150
gooseberries	100	¾ c.	150	150
grapefruit, fresh	100	½ med.	20	70
grapefruit juice, fresh	240	1 c., or 8 oz.	50	75
grapefruit juice, canned	240	1 c., or 8 oz.	50	65
grape juice, canned	100	½ c.	0	20
grapes	100	1 sm. bunch	25	30
guavas	100	1	200	156
haddock	113	4 oz.	7	120
halibut	113	4 oz.	0	120
ham	113	4 oz.	0	800
heart, beef	113	4 oz.	..	660
herring	113	4 oz.	200	120
hominy, white	100	½ c.	0	54
honey	25	1 T.	0	0
huckleberries	100	½ c.	100	45
ice cream, commercial	100	½ c.	170	36
jams	50	4 t.	0	0
jellies	50	4 t.	0	0

[1] Fortified flour means that iron, thiamin, niacin, and sometimes calcium and riboflavin, have been added to refined flour.

VITAMINS			CALCIUM MILLI-GRAMS	PHOSPHO-RUS MILLI-GRAMS	IRON MILLI-GRAMS	PROTEIN GRAMS	CALORIES
RIBOFLAVIN GAMMAS	ASCORBIC ACID MIL-LIGRAMS	D UNITS					
220	0	0	270	90	3.3	10	354
54	0	0	20	90	1	10	354
160	0	0	45	423	5	12	361
..	0	0	7	117	1.6	14	244
0	0	0	0	17	..	8	34
0	0	0	0	0	0	0	90
..	0	0	10	175	2.4	22	153
..	25	0	40	50	0.4	1	37
60	45	0	21	20	0.2	0	36
144	108	0	42	40	0.4	1	72
144	72	0	42	40	0.4	1	100
20	0	0	11	10	0.3	0	60
24	3	0	19	35	0.7	1	80
105	125	0	15	16	3	1	56
198	0	..	18	197	0.5	17	72
222	0	..	20	200	1	19	121
225	0	0	13	54	5.7	20	248
900	4	0	12	129	3.7	17	96
330	0	..	23	246	0.6	19	394
0	0	0	12	112	0	0	355
0	1	0	0	6	0.1	0	101
21	8	0	25	20	0.2	1	60
150	0	2	202	74	0.6	2	208
—	0	0	—	—	—	0	176
—	0	0	—	—	—	0	156

FOOD	WEIGHT, GRAMS	MEASURE	VITAMINS A UNITS	THIAMIN GAMMAS
jello [1]	200	¾ c.	0	0
kale, cooked	100	½ c.	20,000	189
ketchup, tomato	20	1 T.	—	..
kidney, beef	113	4 oz.	1100	300
kohlrabi	100	½ c.	..	30
lamb chop	113	2 chops	0	300
lamb, roast	113	4 oz.	0	225
lamb's-quarters (greens)	100	½ c.	19,000	180
lard	30	2 T.	2	51
leeks	100	½ c.	20	150
lemon juice	50	4 T.	0	24
lentils, cooked	100	½ c.	200	378
lettuce, green	100	10 leaves	2000	75
lettuce, white	100	¼ head	125	51
lime juice	50	¼ c.	65	..
liver, beef	113	4 oz. or 1 sl.	9000	300
liver, calf	113	4 oz. or 1 sl.	7000	250
liver, chicken	113	4 oz. or ½ c.	8000	210
liver, lamb	113	4 oz. or 1 sl.	9000	300
liver, pork	113	4 oz. or 1 sl.	6000	450
lobster, canned	100	½ c.	..	150
loganberries, canned	100	1 c.	..	33
macaroni, white, cooked	100	¾ c.	0	5
macaroni, whole wheat	100	¾ c.	0	410
malted milk, dry	30	2 T.	2040	330

[1] Made with water

RIBOFLAVIN GAMMAS	ASCORBIC ACID MILLIGRAMS	D UNITS	CALCIUM MILLIGRAMS	PHOSPHORUS MILLIGRAMS	IRON MILLIGRAMS	PROTEIN GRAMS	CALORIES
0	0	0	0	0	0	2	112
570	96	0	195	67	2.5	4	45
..	—	0	3	8	0.2	—	21
2520	10	0	9	182	4.2	15	137
120	50	0	195	60	0.7	2	32
330	0	0	21	180	3.3	20	359
320	0	0	21	180	1.7	22	225
600	82	0	180	70	2.6	4	55
9	0	0	0	0	0	0	270
..	24	0	58	56	0.6	2	40
2	25	0	11	6	0.3	0	20
390	0	0	20	77	1.7	9	115
150	7	0	49	28	1.5	1	10
62	5	0	17	40	0.5	1	10
..	18	0	28	17	—	0	20
2500	30	20	11	368	9.2	20	140
2250	25	20	8	420	9.4	23	148
..	25	15	..	..	..	20	130
2500	20	17	8	400	7.9	20	120
2500	12	24	10	370	8.1	20	150
156	5	..	18	188	0.9	16	84
..	35	0	35	24	1.3	1	64
0	0	0	24	119	0.1	3	130
160	0	0	45	423	5.1	4	130
200	0	0	..	..	..	2	82

FOOD	WEIGHT, GRAMS	MEASURE	VITAMINS	
			A UNITS	THIAMIN GAMMAS
mandarin (orange)	100	2 sm.	150	80
margarine	28	1 oz.	.. [1]	0
marmalade, orange	25	1 T.	..	0
mayonnaise	15	1 T.	—	..
melon, cantaloupe	150	½ sm.	900	90
melon, honey dew	150	¼ med.	100	..
melon, watermelon	300	1 med. ser.	450	180
milk, condensed	100	½ c.	680	96
milk, dried, skim	60	5 T.	0	340
milk, evaporated	100	½ c.	680	56
milk, fresh, dry feed	960	1 qt.	800	240
milk, fresh, green feed	960	1 qt.	3500	600
milk, fresh, skim	960	1 qt.	30	300
milk, fresh, whole, average	960	1 qt.	2920	300
milk, goat	960	1 qt.	1630	547
molasses, blackstrap	20	1 T.	0	49
molasses, blackstrap, fortified [2]	20	1 T.	0	1049
molasses, dark, un-refined	20	1 T.	0	0
molasses, light (corn syrup)	20	1 T.	0	0
muffin, bran	35	1 lg.	20	150
muffin, wheat-germ [3]	35	1 lg.	25	450
mushrooms	100	¾ c.	0	160
mustard greens, cooked	100	½ c.	11,000	138

[1] Present if the vitamin is added
[2] Fortified by adding 30 milligrams of thiamin to a pint of molasses
[3] 1 T. per muffin

VITAMINS			CALCIUM MILLI-GRAMS	PHOSPHO-RUS MILLI-GRAMS	IRON MILLI-GRAMS	PROTEIN GRAMS	CALORIES
RIBOFLAVIN GAMMAS	ASCORBIC ACID MIL-LIGRAMS	D UNITS					
150	46	0	45	21	0.5	0	61
0	0	..[1]	—	3	0.1	—	261
..	0	0	8	3	0.1	—	85
7	0	0	2	—	—	—	100
100	50	0	32	30	0.5	1	44
..	90	0	..	..	..	0	35
84	22	0	33	9	0.6	0	90
420	0	0	300	235	0.3	9	326
1625	0	0	1220	850	1.2	34	350
390	0	34[2]	250	200	0.5	8	150
1500	2	0	1100	930	1.6	33	660
2100	12	40	1220	960	2.8	33	660
1925	11	0	1220	960	2.4	34	370
1900	10	20	1200	930	2.2	33	660
950	12	..	1152	960	2	32	672
58	0	0	259	35	9.6	1	52
58	0	0	259	35	9.6	1	52
0	0	0	40	8	1.4	—	57
0	0	0	2	1	0	0	59
40	0	0	26	24	0.4	1	120
62	0	0	26	24	0.6	1	120
70	2	..	14	98	0.7	4	36
450	125	0	291	84	9.1	2	25

[1] If vitamin is added
[2] If irradiated

FOOD	WEIGHT, GRAMS	MEASURE	VITAMINS	
			A UNITS	THIAMIN GAMMAS
mutton, leg	113	4 oz.	0	360
oatmeal, cooked	20	½ c.	0	190
okra	100	½ c.	440	126
olives, green	25	5	50	0
olive oil	15	1 T.	0	0
onions, dry	100	2 sm.	0	42
onions, fresh	100	4 med.	60	42
orange	100	1 med.	190	90
orange juice, canned	240	1 c. or 8 oz.	460	225
orange, fresh	240	1 c. or 8 oz.	460	200
oysters	100	7 med.	250	225
parsley	50	½ c.	8000	57
parsnips	100	½ c.	100	120
peaches, dried	25	3 halves	1000	20
peaches, white, raw	100	3 halves	100	25
peaches, yellow, canned	100	2 lg. halves	600	24
peaches, yellow, raw	100	1 lg.	1000	25
peanut butter	34	2 T.	120	210
peanuts	20	18 nuts	70	225
pears	100	1 med.	17	30
peas, dried, cooked	20	½ c.	520	142
peas, fresh, cooked	100	½ c.	1500	390
pecans	33	10 lg.	90	100
peppers, green	100	1 med.	700	25
peppers, pimiento	100	2 med.	500	..
persimmon, Japanese	150	1 lg.	1600	..
pickles, cucumber	30	4 sm.	0	0

VITAMINS			CALCIUM MILLIGRAMS	PHOSPHORUS MILLIGRAMS	IRON MILLIGRAMS	PROTEIN GRAMS	CALORIES
RIBOFLAVIN GAMMAS	ASCORBIC ACID MILLIGRAMS	D UNITS					
330	0	0	10	270	3	20	191
75	0	0	4	79	1.4	4	80
..	17	0	72	62	2.1	2	24
0	0	0	40	4	0.6	—	35
0	0	0	0	0	0	0	135
125	2	0	41	47	0.3	1	45
125	7	0	41	47	0.4	1	42
75	50	0	44	18	0.4	—	50
230	80	0	90	45	0.9	1	110
230	120	0	90	45	0.9	1	110
540	3	5	33	156	5.8	6	50
..	70	0	23	15	9.6	20	24
..	40	0	60	76	1.7	2	65
50	0	0	12	19	0.6	1	77
65	6	0	10	19	0.2	1	50
60	8	0	10	19	0.3	1	50
65	9	0	10	19	0.3	1	50
200	0	0	24	132	0.6	9	203
110	0	0	15	73	0.4	5	110
60	4	0	15	18	0.3	0	60
162	0	0	17	80	2.8	12	173
250	20	0	28	127	2	7	100
75	0	0	29	112	0.8	3	229
25	125	0	12	28	0.4	1	25
..	200	0	6	26	0.4	1	23
..	40	0	22	21	0.2	2	116
0	0	0	3	2	0.4	0	26

FOOD	WEIGHT, GRAMS	MEASURE	VITAMINS	
			A UNITS	THIAMIN GAMMAS
pie, apple [1]	100	1 lg. sl.	45	18
pie, apricot [1]	100	1 lg. sl.	3700	18
pineapple, canned	100	2 sl.	25	75
pineapple, fresh	100	⅔ c.	30	100
pineapple juice, canned	240	1 c. or 8 oz.	60	105
plums	100	3 med.	130	120
potatoes, sweet	100	1 med.	3600	155
potatoes, white, baked	100	1 med.	0	200
potatoes, white, raw	100	1 med.	0	220
potatoes, yam	100	1 med.	5000	180
pork chops	113	4 oz. or 2 chops	0	540
pork chops, lean, cooked	113	4 oz.	0	800
pork sausage	113	6 links	0	445
prunes, dried	50	6 med.	1500	75
pumpkin	100	½ c.	2500	56
rabbit	113	4 oz.	0	33
radishes	100	15 lg.	0	30
raisins, seeded	30	¼ c.	30	24
raspberries, fresh	100	½ c.	260	21
red-palm oil [2]	15	1 T.	50,000	0
rhubarb	100	½ c.	650	24
rice, brown, cooked	30	¾ c.	20	190
rice, polished, cooked	30	¾ c.	0	0
rice, puffed	10	½ c.	0	—

[1] ⅛ c. fruit in a slice
[2] Imported from India and Africa for making soaps and candles

76

	VITAMINS		CALCIUM MILLI-GRAMS	PHOSPHO-RUS MILLI-GRAMS	IRON MILLI-GRAMS	PROTEIN GRAMS	CALORIES
RIBOFLAVIN GAMMAS	ASCORBIC ACID MIL-LIGRAMS	D UNITS					
25	2	0	8	39	0.2	3	274
50	3	0	11	45	0.4	3	274
25	10	0	8	26	0.1	0	65
25	38	0	8	26	0.2	0	57
60	25	0	20	69	0.2	0	129
56	5	0	20	27	0.5	1	80
150	25	0	19	45	0.9	3	130
75	20	0	13	53	1.5	3	92
75	33	0	13	53	1.5	3	90
360	6	0	44	50	1.1	2	150
312	0	0	16	180	2.5	14	340
225	0	0	18	180	5.7	23	240
300	0	0	7	116	1.6	10	402
325	4	0	27	57	1.5	2	173
57	8	0	23	50	0.9	1	27
72	0	0	20	201	0.6	20	192
54	25	0	21	29	0.9	1	22
50	0	0	20	44	0.9	1	105
. .	30	0	41	38	0.8	1	45
0	0	0	0	0	0	0	100
24	12	0	48	18	0.5	1	20
75	0	0	22	112	1.6	4	117
0	0	0	3	33	0.2	2	117
0	0	0	1	9	0.1	1	35

FOOD	WEIGHT, GRAMS	MEASURE	VITAMINS	
			A UNITS	THIAMIN GAMMAS
rutabagas	100	¾ c.	25	75
salsify (oysterplant)	100	2 roots	0	..
sardines, canned	50	4	200	90
sauerkraut	100	¾ c.	20	8
salmon, canned	113	4 oz.	250	160
scallops	113	4 oz.	..	..
shredded wheat	30	1 biscuit	0	450
shrimp	30	6 med.	25	90
soybeans, dried, cooked	100	½ c.	10	525
soybeans, dried, un-cooked	100	½ c.	25	1312
spaghetti, white, cooked	100	¾ c.	0	5
spaghetti, whole wheat, cooked	100	¾ c.	0	410
spinach, cooked	100	½ c.	11,000	90
squash, Hubbard, cooked	100	½ c.	4000	50
squash, summer, cooked	100	½ c.	1000	40
steak, beef	113	4 oz.	40	150
strawberries, fresh	100	½ c.	100	25
sugar, brown	12	1 T.	0	0
sugar, white, refined	12	1 T.	0	0
syrup, maple	25	1 T.	0	0
sweetbreads, beef	113	4 oz.	..	330
tangerine	100	2 med.	300	120
tapioca, cooked	30	½ c.	0	0
tea, liquid	200	1 c.	0	0

VITAMINS			CALCIUM MILLIGRAMS	PHOSPHORUS MILLIGRAMS	IRON MILLIGRAMS	PROTEIN GRAMS	CALORIES
RIBOFLAVIN GAMMAS	ASCORBIC ACID MILLIGRAMS	D UNITS					
120	26	0	74	56	0.7	1	36
..	7	0	60	53	1.2	3	78
370	0	*	170	195	1	13	103
..	5	0	45	29	0.3	2	28
100	0	440	26	250	1.2	22	203
..	3	..	115	338	3.0	16	81
130	0	0	15	141	1.5	3	108
65	2	5	32	78	0.9	8	27
300	0	0	104	300	4	20	108
750	0	0	260	750	10.1	51	270
0	0	0	25	26	0.2	3	127
160	0	0	45	423	5.1	4	127
312	30	0	78	46	2.5	2	25
75	3	0	19	15	0.5	1	46
50	3	0	18	15	0.3	1	15
250	0	0	12	222	3.4	21	156
..	50	0	34	28	0.6	1	30
0	0	0	15	2	0.4	0	50
0	0	0	0	0	0	0	50
0	0	0	25	4	0.8	0	64
510	0	0	15	595	1.6	14	310
54	48	0	42	17	0.2	1	42
40	0	0	7	30	0.5	—	118
0	0	0	0	0	0	0	0

FOOD	WEIGHT, GRAMS	MEASURE	VITAMINS A UNITS	THIAMIN GAMMAS
tomatoes, canned	100	½ c.	1000	75
tomatoes, fresh	100	1 med.	1500	110
tomato juice, canned	240	8 oz.	3700	195
tongue, beef	113	4 oz.	..	285
turnips, cooked	100	½ c.	0	62
turnips, raw	100	1 med.	0	65
turnip tops, cooked	100	½ c.	11,000	60
tuna, canned	30	¼ c.	20	30
turkey	113	4 oz.	0	150
veal chops	113	4 oz. or 2 chops	0	227
veal, cutlets	113	4 oz.	0	160
veal, leg, cooked	113	4 oz.	0	120
walnuts, black	30	¼ c.	40	110
walnuts, English	30	¼ c.	30	130
watercress	25	¾ c.	1250	30
wheatena, cooked	20	½ c.	7	290
wheat germ	100	½ c.	400	2600
white fish	113	4 oz.	..	120
yeast, bakers', fresh	15	1 cake	0	550
yeast, brewers', dried [1]	15	1 T., 30 tablets	0	2250

[1] Varies widely

VITAMINS			CALCIUM MILLI-GRAMS	PHOSPHO-RUS MILLI-GRAMS	IRON MILLI-GRAMS	PROTEIN GRAMS	CALORIES
RIBOFLAVIN GAMMAS	ASCORBIC ACID MIL-LIGRAMS	D UNITS					
50	20	0	10	29	0.5	1	25
50	25	0	11	29	0.4	1	20
125	48	0	21	38	1	2	48
264	0	0	8	200	6	16	226
62	22	0	56	47	0.5	1	33
62	30	0	56	47	0.6	1	33
450	130	0	347	49	3.4	2	28
..	0	45	10	99	0.5	9	64
240	0	0	30	420	4.5	24	153
298	0	0	12	220	2.8	19	209
360	0	0	15	228	3	20	184
400	0	0	16	240	3	23	180
..	0	0	..	..	2	0	222
..	0	0	22	100	0.5	5	197
90	15	0	40	11	0.8	0	6
30	0	0	10	77	1.1	2	73
750	0	0	71	1050	7.5	24	220
..	0	..	25	263	0.4	22	150
300	0	0	2	74	—	2	20
1000	0	0	11	301	0.9	3	22

SUMMARY OF BODY REQUIREMENTS

Vitamin A

Solubility: in fat, therefore stored if any excess is taken.

Stability: destroyed by oxygen, especially during long cooking; destruction of carotene roughly proportional to loss of color.

Includes: carotene, or provitamin A, a yellow color found in the vegetable kingdom; primary vitamin A, colorless, from animal sources.

Possible toxicity: apparently is not toxic, even when massive doses are taken over long periods.

Suggested daily requirement in units per pound of ideal body weight:

Infants	Children	Adults
300	200	150

Vitamin-B Complex

Solubility: in water, therefore not stored in the body; lost in perspiration and urine.

Stability: thiamin is harmed in cooking; all are partially lost in water in which foods are soaked or cooked if it is thrown away.

Includes: at least ten vitamins and perhaps more; action of these factors may be interdependent. The entire complex can be supplied only by natural sources. Vitamins known chemically: vitamin B_1, thiamin, or thiamin chloride; vitamin B_2, or G, riboflavin; vitamin B_6, pyridoxin; niacin, or niacin acid amide; pantothenic acid; para amino benzoic acid; inositol; biotin; cholin.

Possible toxicity: apparently never toxic if given in the form of the complex; amounts not needed are thrown off in the urine.

Suggested daily requirement of thiamin in gammas per pound of ideal body weight, this amount being used as an index of the entire complex:

Infants	Children	Adults
50	40	35

APPENDIX

Suggested requirements of riboflavin in milligrams per person per day:

Infants	Children	Adults
2	3–4	4–5

Ascorbic acid

Solubility: in water, therefore not stored; lost in perspiration and urine.

Stability: easily destroyed, especially during storage and cooking; lost in water if the water in which foods are soaked or cooked is thrown away.

Chemical name: ascorbic acid.

Possible toxicity: apparently never toxic; when massive doses are taken, excess not needed is thrown off in the urine.

Suggested daily requirement in milligrams of ascorbic acid per pound of ideal body weight:

Infants	Children	Adults
10	3	2

Vitamin D

Solubility: in fat, therefore stored in body, but to limited extent.

Stability: not harmed by cooking or storage.

Possible toxicity: massive doses are sometimes toxic; margin of safety between recommended dose and toxic dose is extremely wide.

Chemical names: viosterol, irradiated ergosterol, calciferol.

Sources: fish-liver oils; irradiated ergosterol; summer sunshine; vitamin-D milk.

Suggested daily requirement in units per individual:

Infants	Children	Adults
1000	1200	800–1200

Vitamin E

Solubility: in fat, therefore stored in the body if excess is taken.

Stability: not harmed by cooking; destroyed when fat becomes rancid.

Chemical name: alpha-tocopherol.

Possible toxicity: apparently not toxic, even in massive doses.

Sources: wheat germ; wheat-germ oil; egg yolk; lettuce; whole-grain breads and cereals; vegetable oils.

Daily requirement: unknown; daily use of one or two of the above sources in the diet.

Vitamin K

Solubility: in fat, therefore stored if well absorbed.

Stability: not harmed in cooking; destroyed by long exposure to light.

Particular need: cannot be absorbed unless bile is present.

Sources: green leaves; vegetable oils; liver.

Daily requirement: unknown; frequent use of liver and green salads.

Calcium

Sources: milk, buttermilk, cheese, and foods prepared with them.

Storage: in the ends of the long bones if any excess is taken.

Particular need: not well used unless vitamin D is supplied.

Suggested daily requirement in milligrams per individual:

Infants	*Children*	*Adults*
1000	1000	1000

Phosphorus

Sources: milk, buttermilk, cheese; eggs; meats, fish, fowl; whole-grain breads and cereals.

Storage: in the ends of the long bones if any excess is taken and calcium is adequately supplied.

Particular need: not well absorbed or used unless vitamin D is supplied.

Suggested daily requirements in milligrams per individual:

Infants	*Children*	*Adults*
930	1000–1500	1500

Iron

Sources well utilized: liver, kidney, heart, muscle meats; black molasses; egg yolk; whole-grain breads and cereals; dried fruits.

Suggested daily requirement in milligrams per individual:

Infants	*Children*	*Adults*
12	20	men 20
		women 25

Copper

Sources: black molasses; liver; nuts; egg yolk; sea foods; legumes; dried fruits; whole-grain breads and cereals; chocolate.

Daily requirement: unknown; daily use of two of the above sources in the diet.

Iodine

Sources: iodized salt; sea foods, ocean fish.

Suggested daily requirement: continual use of iodized salt; sea foods or ocean fish once each week.

Sodium and Chlorine

Source: ordinary table salt.

Suggested daily need: one to two teaspoonfuls per day.

Condition where amount should be increased: in extremely hot weather.

Protein

Proteins of high biological value: essential for growth and maintenance of life; found in milk, eggs, cheese, meats, fish, soybeans, and nuts.

Proteins of medium or low biological value: inadequate to support growth alone; found in corn, legumes, cereals, gelatin.

Suggested daily requirement in grams:

Infants	*Children*	*Adults*
1.5–2 per pound	(1–9 years) 40–70	70–80
	girls (13–20 years) 75–80	
	boys (13–20 years) 85–100	

Calories

Calorie intake must vary with: body weight; age; growth; exercise or physical work; temperature.

Suggested daily requirement in calories per pound of ideal weight:

Infants	*Children*	*Adults*
45	20–30	20, physical work
		15, sedentary work
		8–12, reducing

The ideal weight for 30 years should be maintained throughout life. In the following tables, the **middle** figures give the average weight for medium build. The upper figures are for slender build. The lower figures are for persons having large frames.

Women

Ft.	In.	15 Yr.	20 Yr.	25 Yr.	30 Yr.
		90	95	97	100
4	8	100	105	108	111
		113	117	122	125
		91	96	99	102
4	9	101	107	110	113
		114	119	124	127
		92	98	101	104
4	10	102	109	112	115
		115	123	126	129
		94	100	103	105
4	11	104	111	114	117
		117	125	128	132
		96	103	104	107
5	0	107	114	116	119
		120	128	131	134
		99	105	107	110
5	1	110	117	119	122
		122	132	134	137
		102	108	111	113
5	2	113	120	123	125
		127	135	138	141
		104	111	113	116
5	3	116	123	126	129
		131	138	142	145
		108	113	116	119
5	4	120	126	129	132
		135	142	145	149
		112	117	120	123
5	5	124	130	133	136
		140	146	149	153
		115	121	123	126
5	6	128	134	137	140
		144	151	154	158
		119	124	127	130
5	7	132	138	141	144
		149	155	158	162
		122	127	131	133
5	8	136	141	145	148
		153	159	163	167
		126	131	134	136
5	9	140	145	149	151
		158	163	167	170
		131	134	137	140
5	10	145	149	152	155
		163	168	171	174
		135	139	140	143
5	11	150	154	156	159
		168	173	176	179

Men

Ft.	In.	15 Yr.	20 Yr.	'25 Yr.	30 Yr.
		92	101	105	109
4	11	102	112	117	121
		114	126	131	136
		94	103	107	111
5	0	104	114	119	123
		117	128	134	138
		96	105	109	113
5	1	107	117	121	125
		120	131	136	140
		99	108	112	115
5	2	110	120	124	128
		124	135	139	144
		102	111	115	118
5	3	113	123	128	131
		127	138	144	147
		105	114	119	122
5	4	117	127	132	135
		131	143	148	152
		109	118	123	125
5	5	121	131	136	139
		136	147	153	156
		113	122	126	129
5	6	125	135	140	143
		140	152	157	161
		116	125	130	132
5	7	129	139	144	147
		145	156	162	165
		120	129	133	136
5	8	133	143	148	151
		149	161	166	170
		123	132	137	141
5	9	137	147	152	156
		154	165	171	175
		128	136	141	145
5	10	142	151	157	161
		159	170	176	181
		132	141	146	150
5	11	147	156	162	167
		165	175	182	188
		137	145	151	156
6	0	152	161	168	173
		171	181	189	194
		141	150	157	161
6	1	157	166	174	179
		176	186	195	201
		146	154	161	167
6	2	162	171	179	185
		182	192	201	208

First, estimate your ideal weight. Use this weight in making your calculations.

Vitamin A: ideal weight × 150 units per pound = daily need.

Vitamin-B complex: ideal weight × 30 gammas of thiamin per pound = daily need.

Riboflavin: 4 milligrams, or 4000 gammas, daily.

Ascorbic acid: ideal weight × 2 milligrams per pound = daily need.

Vitamin D: 800–1200 units daily. May be omitted from June until September if you get fifteen minutes of sunshine daily between 10 A.M. and 2 P.M., or several hours of sunshine one day each week.

Vitamin E: eat one or two foods daily which are rich in this vitamin.

Calcium: 1000 milligrams daily.

Phosphorus: 1500 milligrams daily.

Iron: 20–25 milligrams daily.

Copper: eat two foods daily which are rich in this mineral.

Iodine: daily use of iodized salt.

Protein: 70–80 grams daily. Should be largely protein of high biological value.

Calories: ideal weight × 12, 15, or 20 calories per pound = daily need. Except when gaining or reducing is desired, calories need not be calculated.

Compare the amounts of each factor you need for full health with those you have actually eaten, as in the example given on pages **88-89**.

Example:

Helen H., 17 years old. Actual weight 130; ideal weight 120. Her ideal requirements for a day are as follows:

Vitamin A:	120 × 150 = 18,000 units.
Thiamin:	120 × 30 = 3600 gammas.
Riboflavin:	4 milligrams, or 4000 gammas.
Ascorbic acid:	120 × 2 = 240 milligrams.
Vitamin D:	1200 units.
Calcium:	1000 milligrams.
Phosphorus:	1500 milligrams.
Iron:	25 milligrams.
Protein:	80 grams.
Calories:	120 × 15 = 1800

The following table is an analysis of foods eaten in one day by Helen H., age 17 years. If her diet is to be adequate, it must supply each requirement in the amount computed on page 87. With the exception of calories, excess over these amounts is advantageous, especially in the case of calcium, iron, and all vitamins.

FOOD	MEASURE	VITAMINS	
		A UNITS	THIAMIN GAMMAS
Breakfast			
apricots, dried..............	8 halves	6850	48
wheat-germ cereal............	½ c.	400	2600
milk, evaporated.............	¼ c.	340	28
toast, whole wheat...........	1 sl.	10	180
butter......................	1 t.	112	6
milk, skim..................	1 gl.	7	75
Midmorning			
orange......................	1 med.	190	90
Lunch			
cheese omelet			
egg.......................	1 av.	600	65
cheese, American...........	1-in. cube	500	19
milk, skim................	¼ c.	—	18
lettuce and tomato salad			
lettuce, green.............	5 leaves	1000	37
tomato....................	1 med.	1500	110
mayonnaise................	1 t.	—	0
milk, skim..................	1 gl.	7	75
grapefruit...................	½ med.	20	70
Midafternoon			
milk, skim..................	1 gl.	7	75
molasses, blackstrap..........	1 T.	0	49
Dinner			
tomato-juice cocktail.........	1 gl.	3700	195
liver, pork..................	1 sl.	6000	450
beet greens.................	½ c.	22,000	100
carrots.....................	½ c., diced	4500	70
peach-cheese salad			
peach, yellow, canned........	½ lg.	300	12
cottage cheese.............	1 T.	22	2
lettuce, green.............	2 leaves	400	14
milk, skim..................	1 gl.	7	75
cantaloupe..................	½ sm.	900	90
At bedtime			
orange......................	1 med.	190	90
fish-liver-oil capsule..........	1	10,000	0
Total for entire day....................		59,562	4643
Helen's daily requirements for full health...........		18,000	3600

Planned Nutrition

Since Helen's present weight is 130 and her ideal weight 120, she is eating slightly less than her normal calorie intake. In order to avoid excess weight, she drinks skim milk rather than whole milk and eats bread only at breakfast.

	VITAMINS						
RIBO-FLAVIN GAMMAS	ASCORBIC ACID MILLI-GRAMS	D UNITS	CALCIUM MILLI-GRAMS	PHOS-PHORUS MILLI-GRAMS	IRON MILLI-GRAMS	PROTEIN GRAMS	CALORIES
250	0	0	16	30	0.8	1	102
750	0	0	71	1050	7.5	24	220
195	0	17 [1]	125	100	0.2	4	75
100	0	0	22	102	1.1	3	75
0	0	2	0	0	0	0	38
480	2	0	305	240	0.6	8	92
75	50	0	44	18	0.4	—	50
150	0	50	32	112	1.5	6	70
100	0	0	190	137	0.2	6	80
120	0	0	76	60	0.1	2	24
75	3	0	25	14	0.7	0	5
50	25	0	11	29	0.4	1	20
—	0	0	0	—	—	—	33
480	2	0	305	240	0.6	8	92
60	45	0	21	20	0.2	0	36
480	2	0	305	240	0.6	8	92
58	0	0	259	35	9.6	1	52
125	48	0	21	38	1.0	2	48
2500	12	24	10	370	8.1	20	150
500	50	0	94	40	3.2	2	28
75	5	0	45	41	0.6	1	30
30	4	0	5	10	0.1	0	25
40	0	—	122	40	0	2	12
30	—	0	10	4	—	0	1
480	2	0	305	240	0.6	8	92
100	50	0	32	30	0.5	1	44
75	50	0	44	18	0.4	—	50
0	0	1200	0	0	0	0	6
7378	350	1293	2495	3258	39	108	1642
4000	240	1200	1000	1500	25	80	1800

[1] If irradiated

INDEX

THESE PAGES ARE TO BE USED FOR NOTES,
SPECIAL RECIPES AND DIET CHARTS

For Complete Catalog
of Natural Health Literature
send $1.00 to
BENEDICT LUST PUBLICATIONS
The Original Health Book People
P.O. Box 404
New York, N.Y. 10156-0404